Rebalance your metabolism

IN 21 DAYS

- THE ORIGINAL -

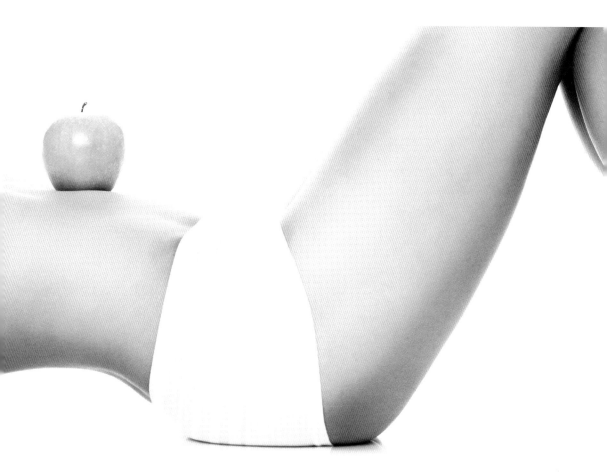

Arno Schikowsky I Rudolf Binder MD I Christian Mörwald

LEGAL NOTICE

This handbook was compiled by:
Arno Schikowsky, a.schikowsky@21tage.info
Hochstrasser Weg 2a, 83064 Raubling

Authors:
Arno Schikowsky, a.schikowsky@21tage.info
Rudolf Binder MD, www.drbinder.lnfo
Christian Mörwald, cmoerwald@t-online.de

Translation:
From the original German by
Andrea Campbell & Deborah Middleton,
andrea_campbell@gmx.net

Disclaimer:
The contents of this handbook are for information purposes only. We neither recommend nor promote the methods mentioned in this book. Procedures or advice are based on personal experiences only. The contents neither claim to be complete nor can their topicality, accuracy or balance of information presented be guaranteed. The contents of this book are not a substitute for the professional advice of a medical doctor or pharmacist. Under no circumstances may the contents be the basis for the independent modification or termination of a treatment for an illness or diagnosis. In the event of health questions or complaints please always consult a medical doctor. The authors do not assume any liability for any inconvenience or damage caused while carrying out the metabolic diet and the information presented in this handbook.

Design & Production:
Kainz Werbe GmbH, Kolbermoor
1. Edition 2015, Printed in Germany

Images and photographic material: © by www.fotolia.com
p. 1: © Kalim; p. 8: © drubig-photo; p. 15: © Artem Furman;
p. 18: © Subbotina Anna; p. 22: © Fisher Photostudio;
p. 25: © Leonid & Anna Dedukh; p. 27: © Warren Goldswain;
p. 28: © racamani; p. 30: © PhotoSG; p. 33: © underdogstudios;
p. 34: © Marina Lohrbach; p. 36/43: © opolja; p. 39: © Adam Gregor;
p. 44: © monticellllo; p. 46: © fotoliaxrender; p. 50: © ag visuell;
p. 52: © Lonely; p. 54: © mimagephotos; p. 56: © Natalia Klenova;
p. 59: © Carmen Steiner; p. 60: © charlyblende;
p. 62: © drubig-photo; p. 64: © paul prescott; p. 66: © julief514;
p. 68: © vasilevki; p. 69: © Tijana; p. 70: © Artem Furman;
p. 74: © iko; p. 76: © bonninturina; p. 78: © Grafvision;
p. 84: © Eva Gruendemann; p. 85: © darzel;
p. 87: © Miguel Garcia Saaved; p. 96: © dusk; p. 104: © babsi_w;
p. 125: © karinrin; p. 135: © gitusik; p. 145: © aimy27feb

Sales & Distribution:
Arno Schikowsky, a.schikowsky@21tage.info

US-Edition

Contents

We dedicate this book to our families and the many, many people who have placed their trust in us

The Authors

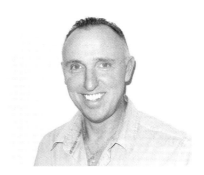

Arno Schikowsky was born in 1965. A former competitive athlete with an education in sports and fitness (ICC), he can look back on 32 years of experience as a fitness and nutrition coach, instructor and sports rehabilitation trainer. He has been the successful founder and owner of a fitness center for 21 years.

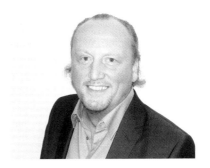

Rudolf Binder MD is a specialist in general medicine, naturopathy and acupuncture. A registered physician with his own practice in Bavaria, South Germany since 1998, he has also worked successfully for many years as a hypnotherapist, Klinghardt® therapist and nutrition coach. With over 20 years of experience, to him the appreciation of a healthy, holistic lifestyle is a matter close to his heart and makes him a sought-after speaker on the subject.

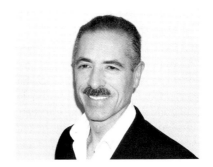

Christian Mörwald was born in 1966 in Bavaria, South Germany. As a professional trainer for sports, health and prevention, he has been intensively involved in nutrition for about 30 years in the area of health and physical performance. As a successful partner and coach in a fitness center, he has a wealth of experience in this field.

Foreword Arno Schikowsky

Dear Reader!

When I first heard about the 21 Day Metabolic Diet – and that was not so very long ago – I rejected this programme outright. For over 30 years I have been studying any and all diets that have come on to the market. I have tried many of the nutritional programmes myself with varying degrees of success. I could not tell you how many clients I have advised over the past few decades. I am sure there were thousands. I gave numerous lectures but did my clients have lasting success? Hardly. In most cases they failed owing to the bad quality of the programme, its suitability to everyday life and, of course, a lack of discipline on their part.

And now another diet? A "new" one that was supposed to outrival all the diets I had known before? A nutrition programme that did not meet caloric requirements, combined with homeopathy and supplements? I thought immediately of muscle loss, the so-called "yo-yo" effect and hunger. And as for homeopathy? For me, at that time, it was complete nonsense. I brushed it off and never gave it another thought. However, weeks later, after I had read more and more success stories, I became curious. The results were so phenomenal that I finally did take a closer look.

Shed a few pounds quickly? Who does not want that? With this book, we – Arno Schikowsky (professional sports and nutrition coach for over 30 years), Rudolf Binder MD (specialist in general medicine and naturopathy) and Christian Mörwald (professional trainer for sports, health and prevention) - introduce you to the 21 Day Metabolic Diet.

This book is intended to help you live a healthier life, to lose weight in a healthy way, without feeling hungry, and all this with an ease you have never known until now.

I am aware that this book will be in the firing line of experts, however, I have used simple language to make it understandable for those people who have little or no dietary knowledge. Homeopathy, micronutrients and a low calorie diet that is suitable for everyday life: This is the "21 Day Metabolic Diet."

We have shown in detail how this new/old "diet" works: step by step with delicious recipes and exercise recommendations. We have also pointed out any possible challenges and given advice regarding nutrition, amongst many other things.

All the information or statements are based on experiences that I have had with my clients. It is quite possible that, to date, there have been no clinical studies or medical proof. However the results speak for themselves.

The "Questions and Answers" section from page 146 onwards will help and support you to rebalance your metabolism. From page 78 onwards, you will find over 100 recipes for delicious meals.

Happy reading!

Arno Schikowsky

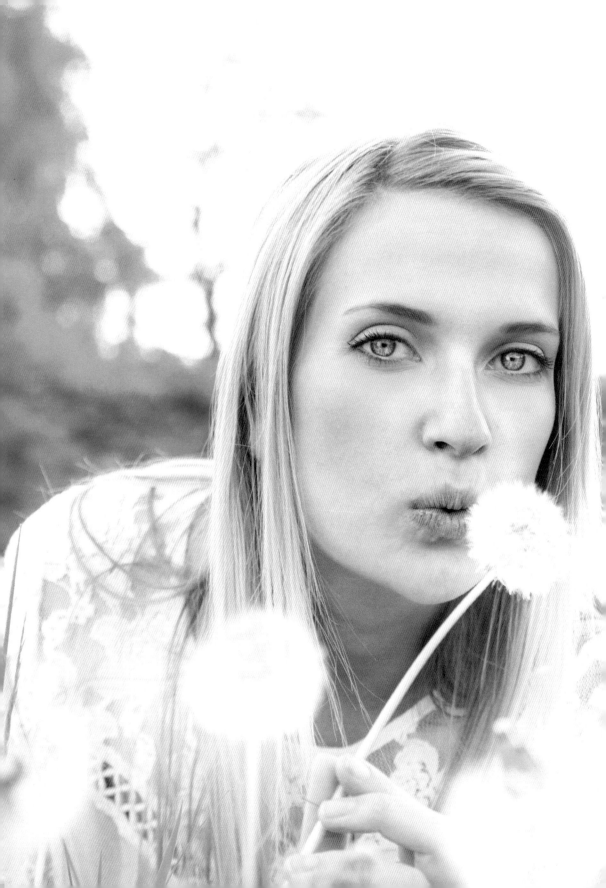

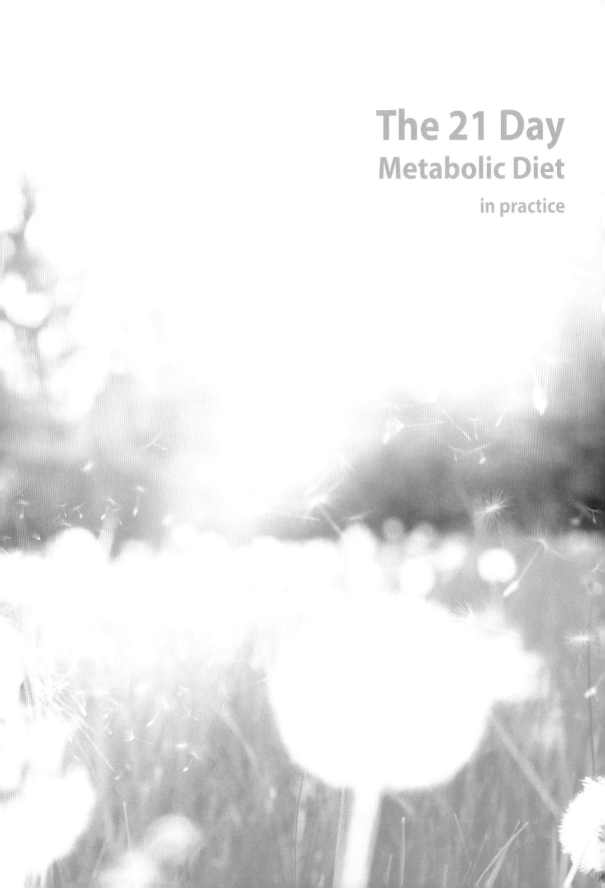

The 21 Day
Metabolic Diet
in practice

The 21 Day Metabolic Diet in practice

For those who want to start right away we have put the "practical part" at the very beginning. For those readers who prefer to familiarize themselves first as to how the rebalancing of the metabolism works, skip this chapter for the moment and continue reading on page 19 before you come back to this section. I highly recommend you read and follow the instructions carefully, because they are crucial for the diet to succeed.

The health benefits of the metabolic diet can be tremendous.

Here are a few results that my clients have achieved in the first few weeks:

➡ Their weight decreased by up to 26 lbs in 21 days

➡ Stubborn body fat could be reduced

➡ They found, however, that structural fat had hardly decreased

➡ They experienced a minimal amount of reduction of muscle mass

➡ In many cases the skin seemed to have improved

➡ Better regulation of the acid/alkaline (pH) balance

➡ Most felt energetic, almost "rejuvenated"

➡ For the most part, there was no "yo-yo" effect

People, who, for health reasons are not sure if the metabolic diet is suitable for them, should consult an experienced medical practitioner. In the event of health issues (such as diabetes or high blood pressure) we advise you to consult with your physician before you begin the diet. You will experience dramatically positive changes that may require an adjustment to the amount of your medication. You and your doctor should be prepared for this. But would it be so bad if you had to take less medication?

On page 153 you will find a summary of the metabolic diet for your attending physician.

The complete metabolic diet comprises 4 phases:

1. The loading phase
   Duration   2 days

2. The actual diet phase
   Duration   minimum 21 days

3. The stabilization phase
   Duration   21 days

4. The test phase
   Duration   6 months

Each of these four phases is equally important for lasting success.

Preparation

Make a decision as to when you want to start. It would be ideal if you chose a fairly quiet time for the diet phase without any extreme physical and mental exertion. On the other hand, there is never a perfect time – so don´t procrastinate too long and get started!

Sports people can and should continue their usual workout. Generally, sport is not a prerequisite for a good result with the diet. However people

NOTE:

A journey of a thousand miles starts with a single step.

who practice sport reduce more body fat because the energy that is needed for their activities has to be provided from their stored fat.

In principle, this diet is not recommended during pregnancy or lactation. Women who are still menstruating achieve best results if they start right after their period. The two days of the loading phase can be carried out during their period.

Please start the diet only when you have all the necessary products to hand.

➡ Activator, nutritional supplements and aspartame free protein powder (source of supply please see p. 154).

➡ Food for the first few days (pre-plan your shopping)

➡ If necessary, buy new kitchen scales, personal scales and a tape measure.

The Start

Very important: jot down your initial weight and motivate yourself during the diet by documenting your success, for example:

➡ Good photos of your body e.g. front, back, side as well as partial view (note the conditions in which you took the shots – your position and the camera position as well as the camera settings)

➡ Determine the size of your waist (measure in the same place each time and make a note)

➡ Always weigh yourself at the same time of day and under the same conditions.

Note: **Your body will not change in a uniform way. Periods of stagnation and fluctuation are absolutely normal.**

The Loading Phase (2 days)

Now you start taking the activator. If possible evenly distributed throughout the day. Before breakfast, lunch and dinner and once more before bedtime. At least 20 minutes before eating, drinking coffee, brushing your teeth or smoking.

Eat what you like, preferably lots of fatty foods and sweet things. I am sure you will have lots of ideas. Just eat as much as you can.

It is important to flood the body with as many calories as possible. Of course, it is quite normal for your weight to increase over these two days. However, in order for the diet to be a success, these two days are critically important.

The Diet Phase

Continue taking the activator as indicated for the loading phase.

This is your dietary plan:

Breakfast	1 portion (1 oz) of aspartame free protein powder made with water
Mid morning snack	1 piece of fruit if desired, max. 3-1/2 oz. **Only if really necessary**
Lunch	4-1/4 oz of protein, cooked weight, with vegetables or salad as much as you like
Afternoon snack	1 piece of fruit if desired, max. 3-1/2 oz. **Only if really necessary**
Dinner	4 oz of protein, cooked weight, with vegetables or salad as much as you want
Snacks	Wasa cracker – max. 1/day or Grissini – max. 2/day
Liquids	At least 2 quarts

Our clients confirmed that they were hardly ever hungry, but rather experienced some cravings, despite the low caloric intake from the food. Our clients believed that the activator contributed to that. During the metabolic diet, stored deposits of fat are dissolved which in turn supply the body with energy.

For readers who prefer to lose body fat as quickly as possible (and I think most of you want that) note, that if you forego the fruit and the cracker/grissini as snacks, you will have better results. By saving these extra calories the body will burn off more stored fat instead.

For the same reason those who want to see fast results should not use skin care products and creams that contain animal and vegetable fats or oils because some of these ingredients will be absorbed by the skin.

You prepare your meals from the following foods

Protein	Meat: filet, steak, beef, lean hamburger meat, roast beef, chicken breast, veal, lean pork, turkey breast and turkey escalope .
	Fish and seafood: gilthead, pike, halibut, flounder, sole, cod, perch, tuna in water, shrimps, prawns, mussels, squid rings, lobster and crab.
	Prepare everything with as little fat as possible, remove any skin and visible fat before preparation. Do not use fat or oil for cooking. E.g. prepare meat on a grill.
Vegetables	Cauliflower, Broccoli, white mushrooms, Belgian endives, Chinese cabbage (Bok choy), kale, white and red cabbage, Savoy cabbage, fennel, spring onions, lettuce, iceberg salad, rocket, Swiss chard, bell pepper, leek, radish, Brussels sprouts, cucumber, sauerkraut, asparagus, tomatoes, spinach, celery, onions and zucchini.
	Everything should be as fresh as possible, frozen vegetables can also be used.
Fruits **Only if absolutely necessary**	Sour apples, oranges, grapefruit, strawberries, pears, blackberries, pomegranates, blueberries, red currants, cherries, tangerines, mangoes, nectarines, passion fruit, peaches, plums, cranberries and gooseberries.
	Please eat them while as fresh as possible.
Spices	Rock salt (Himalayan salt), pepper, mustard powder, garlic, basil, parsley, thyme, marjoram etc. vinegar/balsamic vinegar, cider vinegar, Dijon mustard (without sugar), soy sauce, sambal olek, tabasco, wasabi, cinnamon, lemon juice and stevia to sweeten.
Liquids	Still water (at least 2 quarts/day), coffee black (max. 1 tsp. milk per cup if necessary) and tea (black, green, mate or herbal).

This selection of foods is from the book by
Matthias Jünemann "Die Adipositas Kur", Published by "Books on Demand GmbH, Norderstedt, ISBN 978-3842372320.

During the diet phase only the foods indicated are allowed.
Make the choice to eat good quality, fresh food.
Any food not on the list is strictly forbidden!

Alternative sources of protein for vegetarians and vegans:

Nutritional values of the products	Protein (oz)	Fat (oz)	Carbo-hydrates (oz)	Energy (kcal)
In comparison *4-1/4 oz freshly cooked beef*	*1.27*	*0.15*	*0.00*	*182*
4-1/2 tablespoons Triple Protein Shake	1.34	0.0	0.06	132
3-1/2 oz Harzer cheese or other low fat cheese	1.05	0.02	0.003	125
3-1/2 oz Seitan (wheat protein)	1.34	0.11	0.13	222
7-1/2 cups Soy milk light	1.11	0.63	1.06	390 !
1lb 10-1/2 oz Soy yogurt	1.22	0.70	0.53	383 !
8-3/4 oz Tofu	1.19	0.66	0.16	322 !
7 oz Lopino from lupin protein	1.26	0.23	0.23	230
8-3/4 oz Cottage cheese low fat	1.17	0.12	0.30	203
10-1/2 oz low fat Quark cheese	1.30	0.04	0.41	195
5 cups skim milk	1.20	0.11	1.70	360
7-1/2 tablespoons hemp protein powder	1.29	0.35	0.20	268
10 egg whites	1.26	0.04	0.02	160

Please note the quantities indicated when using alternative types of protein so as to guarantee enough protein. Please also note that some of the alternative sources of protein mentioned may have significantly more fat and/or carbohydrates than the approved protein on p.12, which means more calories, thus slowing down weight loss.

In the recipe section you will find ideas on how to prepare delicious meals.

For packed meals, choose dishes that are easy to take with you and which can be eaten cold (e.g. tuna with tomatoes).

In restaurants it is usually possible to order a piece of grilled meat or fish and a bowl of salad seasoned with herbs and vinegar.

When invited to a friend´s house it is a good idea to speak to your host about your diet beforehand. But it will be noticed anyway!

Role of Micronutrients

Micronutrients, e.g. vitamins, minerals and trace elements are of essential importance to our health. Since you provide your body with less fuel during the metabolic diet and therefore fewer nutrients (because, after all, you want to reduce body fat) and because due to the fat loss your requirements are even higher, it is of utmost importance to supplement with micronutrients.

A lack of micronutrients is often the reason for a susceptibility to infection and other illnesses. An optimal supply of micronutrients can protect you from this. Of course, in theory, it is possible to provide your body with sufficient nutrients if a healthy lifestyle and nutritionally rich diet are guaranteed. However, who nowadays is able to provide their body with first class, freshly harvested, natural, unprocessed foods and furthermore is able to avoid all the negative influences such as environmental pollutants? As a matter of fact, as negative environmental influences increase, the quality of our nutrition takes a nosedive. Our foodstuff actu-

ally contains fewer and fewer nutrients. For example, bananas in 1996 had 45 % fewer nutrients than back in 1985. The research of two-time Nobel Prize winner, Professor Linus Pauling, showed that people from the stone age had 300 % more micronutrients in their diet than what is recommended today by the German Association of Nutrition (DGE) and it is scientifically proven that over half the German population never receives the recommended amount.

People who live stress free and away from harmful environmental influences, who do not smoke or drink alcohol, who exercise regularly and eat 5 daily portions of fresh fruits and vegetables, fresh fish three times a week and lean game once a week, who abstain from sugar, too much salt and fat, who live on a quiet island far away from any pollution, these people will likely not experience the diseases associated with modern day living.

The majority of my clients have reported having had excellent experiences with the first class supplements from Lifeplus (for source of supply see page 154).

This program of supplements from Lifeplus has been tried and tested by my clients:

	Comprehensive vitamin mineral drink with fiber	Organic sulfur	Anti-oxidants*	Omega-3 Fatty acids
Morning	2 scoops	4 tablets	2 tablets	1 capsule
Evening		4 tablets		1 capsule

* For best results: take at least 30 minutes before your meal

Lifeplus products are outstanding, high quality supplements manufactured by cold processing, the finest, natural raw materials, thus ensuring that the potency of the enzymes and vitamins is retained. (Heat would destroy their potency and reduce their nutritional benefits). Furthermore, these products do not contain synthetic fillers as binders. Instead Lifeplus uses a formula made from special herbs, phytonutrients, co-factors, plant enzymes and more than 30 different fruits and vegetables which synergistically assist the body's assimilation of the products' active ingredients. Furthermore, their products contain no artificial additives such as colorants, preservatives, fragrances or flavors (source: www.lifeplus.com).

Should you use different products, the following regime has been tried and tested:

➡ Organic sulfur in the morning and in the evening. Take 1 scoop with still water together with a binder such as Chlorella

➡ Omega-3 fatty acids according to instructions. 1-2 capsules in the morning and in the evening

➡ Vitamins and antioxidants as per the instructions

➡ PH tablets or powder as per the instructions 3 x day after meals

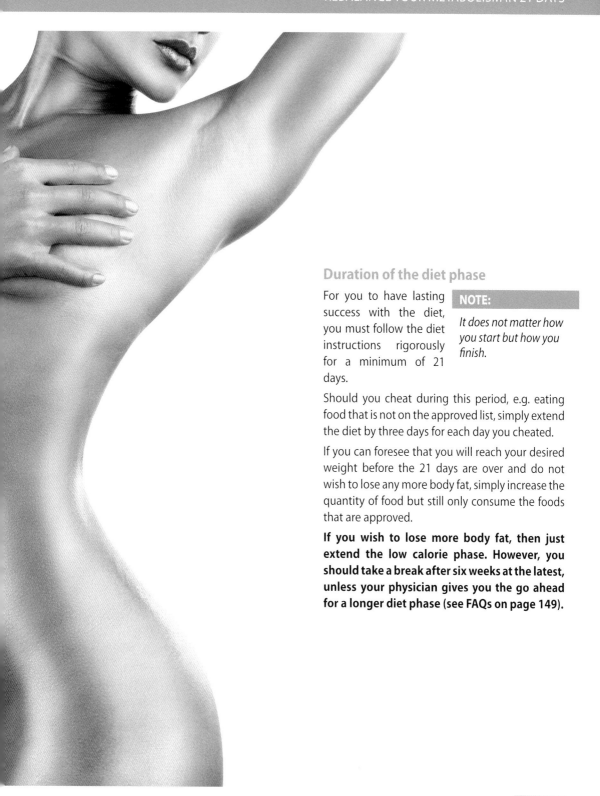

Duration of the diet phase

For you to have lasting success with the diet, you must follow the diet instructions rigorously for a minimum of 21 days.

NOTE:

It does not matter how you start but how you finish.

Should you cheat during this period, e.g. eating food that is not on the approved list, simply extend the diet by three days for each day you cheated.

If you can foresee that you will reach your desired weight before the 21 days are over and do not wish to lose any more body fat, simply increase the quantity of food but still only consume the foods that are approved.

If you wish to lose more body fat, then just extend the low calorie phase. However, you should take a break after six weeks at the latest, unless your physician gives you the go ahead for a longer diet phase (see FAQs on page 149).

The Stabilization Phase

During the stabilization phase your new set-point, your new weight, will be established. This phase is just as important as the low calorie phase. The stabilization phase begins right after the diet phase and takes 21 days. This way the "yo-yo" effect is by all accounts prevented.

Now you no longer take the activator but eat just as before for another two days until the effect of the globules has declined.

Weigh yourself on the morning of the third day. This is your new set point which is supposed to be maintained until the end of the stabilization phase. Small fluctuations of 2 lbs or so are perfectly normal.

Now there are only 19 days left. The globules no longer have any effect. This is why your body now needs to be provided with the necessary fuel from food. Do not eat a low calorie diet anymore. Feelings of hunger will return. Watch your weight. Do not continue losing weight as now you would lose muscle. However, keeping your nutritional plan from the diet phase as a basic structure, you can now increase the amount of protein and also incorporate other healthy proteins (e.g. dairy products, eggs, nuts, legumes). You can also eat more fruit now. Add first class cold pressed oils (e.g. olive oil, linseed oil) to your daily diet. Sugar, floury and processed foods are still a no-no. Also, continue to stay away from carbohydrates such as potatoes, pasta and rice. The same applies for alcoholic beverages. Monitor yourself carefully to see when your body does not tolerate a certain food and then avoid it.

In the recipe section, you will also find ideas and recipes to prepare delicious meals for yourself during the stabilization phase.

In order to guarantee success with your weight loss, we recommend you keep taking nutritional supplements while eating a healthy diet.

This is an example of supplements guaranteeing optimal nutrients from Lifeplus

	Comprehensive vitamin mineral drink with fiber	Organic sulfur* (if desired)	Anti-oxidants	Omega-3 Fatty acids* (if desired)
Morning	2 scoops	4 tablets	2 tablets	1 capsule
Evening		4 tablets		1 capsule

* Your daily needs of organic sulfur are usually met by natural foods such as fresh fruits and vegetables, fresh meat and seafood. Your daily requirements of Omega-3 fatty acids are supplied by oily coldwater fish. If you provide your body with sufficient quantities, supplementing is not absolutely necessary in the stabilization phase for you to be successful with the diet. The other supplements should be taken in the same way as during the diet phase.

TIP:

We recommend you continue with the nutritional supplements in the stabilization phase as described above and do not follow the short version which is also offered and which includes just multivitamin and mineral tablets.

Although both versions work, we have experienced that if the original plan is adopted as described in this book, it is easier to control your weight during the stabilization phase because the fiber at breakfast time ensures a longer lasting feeling of satisfaction, in comparison to the vitamin and mineral tablets alone.

The test phase

In the test phase the main focus is on keeping off the weight you have lost and not falling back into old habits.

During the next 6 months you are encouraged to test more and more items from your personal food choices. Add new foods to your diet and observe exactly how your body reacts to them. Keep your weight in check. You should not stray more than 5 lbs from your set-point.

At first include more vegetables into your daily diet then add more fruit. Different types of bread, potatoes, rice and pasta can now be added as nutritional components. Later on, you may wish to try your favorite "dietary vices" like chocolate, ice cream, cake…).

We recommend for your own good that you keep taking basic nutritional supplements.

This is an example of your daily nutritional supplement requirements with products from Lifeplus

	Multivitamin and minerals	Organic sulfur* (if desired)	Anti-oxidants	Omega-3 Fatty acids* (if desired)
Morning	2 tablets	4 tablets	2 tablets	1 capsule
Midday	2 tablets			
Evening	2 tablets	4 tablets		1 capsule

* Please see note from p. 16

Now what's next?

Do not stray from your (new) habits learned from the metabolic diet. Do not return to your old and unhealthy lifestyle because you have accomplished a lot. Stick to your new lifestyle and your new weight while observing a few important principles:

➜ Make sure you drink plenty of fluids (2 quarts/day minimum) preferably non-carbonated water

➜ Keep your sugar intake low

➜ Avoid unhealthy fats

➜ Make sure you provide your body with sufficient essential fatty acids

➜ Watch your salt consumption

➜ Eat lots of fresh vegetables, salads and fruit

➜ Eat sufficient high quality protein

➜ Reduce your consumption of ready-made meals

➜ Get regular exercise

➜ Avoid "poisons" like nicotine and alcohol

➜ Get enough sleep

➜ Avoid stress or make sure to compensate for it

➜ An optimal supply of micronutrients from nutritional supplements can be very beneficial for your health, wellbeing and performance.

➜ **Note:** Nutritional supplements are not a substitute for natural and healthy food. Your nutrition is the basis of your health. But, in all honesty, who manages to always keep up a healthy way of eating? **It is about supplementing a preferably balanced diet with a specific and ongoing supply of excellent micronutrients.**

➜ Take care of yourself and watch your weight!

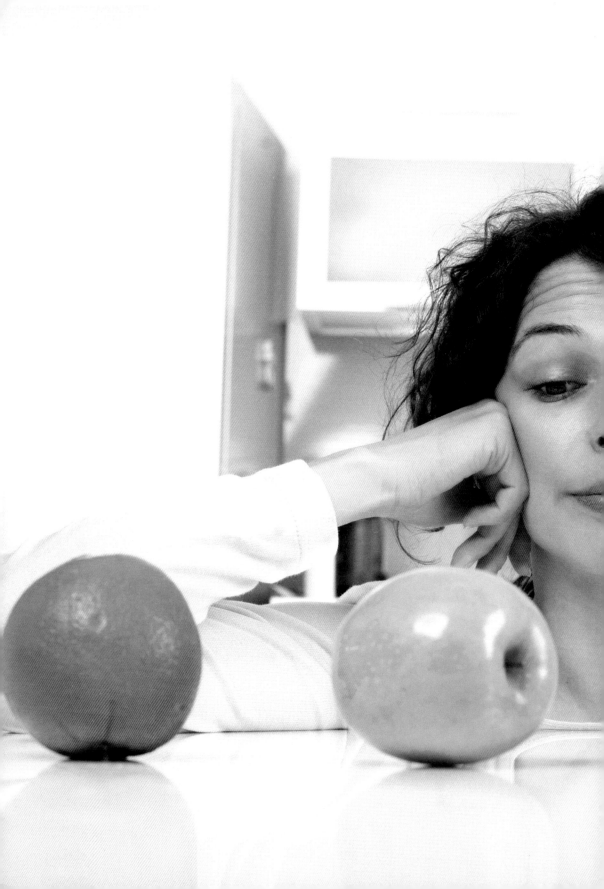

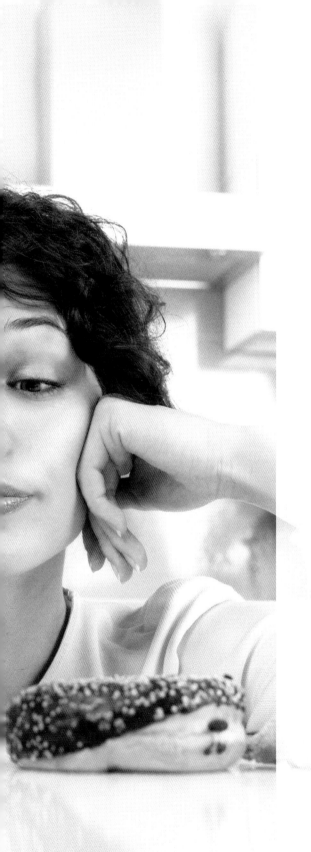

THE 7 PILLARS OF

the 21 Day
Metabolic Diet

21 DAYS – WHY?

by Rudolf Binder MD

THE 7 PILLARS OF THE 21 DAY METABOLIC DIET
by Rudolf Binder MD

21 DAYS – WHY?

It usually starts with you standing in front of the mirror or the closet thinking:

"This pot belly has got to go!" or "This butt no longer fits into these pants!"

After that, come all kinds of diet recommendations, some of them tried and tested others just known from hearsay. Now, well-known, supposedly still unknown, and easy to find weight loss programs all run through your head.

The selection is mostly based on the following criteria:

➡ Fast and effective
➡ Uncomplicated and suitable for everyday life
➡ Sustainable
➡ Revitalizing and maintaining performance
➡ Inexpensive
➡ Healthy
➡ No psychological stress

Welcome to the 21 Day Metabolic Diet!
You have reached your destination!

This metabolic concept is not new, however, it excites so many because it satisfies the above criteria. The protocol has been constantly modified and improved and can look back on millions of experiences of many, many users.

There is no reason to be ashamed if you are pragmatic and say "I couldn´t care less how it works as long as it works!" and just go back to Page 10 and start the diet. Don´t worry! This way, you WILL also be successful!

However, should you like to know, why this "comprehensive protocol" is so surprisingly efficient and if you want to know how you can keep up a healthy lifestyle afterwards and, if you would like to know how you can help and guide others to successfully complete the diet, then set aside a little time during the coming days and weeks.

Leaf through the following pages, maybe when you are in bed, and read about why the 21 Day Metabolic Diet is so successful. Should you already have started the diet, carefully note how your body looks! Maybe you can already see some surprising changes taking place in your metabolism while you are still reading the early chapters.

Why do we need a phase where we consciously influence our metabolism?
An example:

Maybe you remember how you learned to drive. After the introduction about how the car works, it probably would have been best if the driving instructor (or whoever taught you to drive) had said: "Hold the steering wheel firmly with both hands, step on the accelerator and under no circumstances turn the wheel. Just keep going straight, then nothing can happen!"

But he didn´t say that because there are twists and turns which we have to follow if we want to stay on the road. This means, stepping on the gas, braking, shifting gears, and once in a while steering to the left or right simply to follow the road. We want to get to our destination safely, don't we?

Our everyday eating habits are pretty much the same. The dietary rules that we are still given in terms of how often, how much and what we should eat may be helpful for the rest of our lives, if we stick to them. This means during birthdays, weddings and holidays. What fun!

Are you one of those people who, once in a while, like to eat a hamburger or a pizza, a donut or an ice cream? And what about a glass or two of coca cola, wine or beer? Then sticking to these general eating habits is the best way n o t to maintain your weight because there comes a time when you have to compensate for any excess calories. Otherwise these "slip-ups" accumulate and end up on your hips and, for sure, will show up on the scales. When you steer to the right, at some point you will have to steer to the left otherwise you will end up driving in a circle. And as far as your weight is concerned, it can easily end up spiraling out of control. Driving "just straight ahead" is not enough to maintain your weight. We are not saying that you cannot follow the twists and turns of everyday treats, however, you have to counteract them – even if driving in zig zags – in order to arrive at your destination.

The 21 Day Metabolic Diet is a healthy and efficient plan. If your body clearly shows visible effects caused by the "slip-ups" of the past few years, then this is the right choice for a new beginning. If you cheat just once in a while in the future, all you need to do is simply practice a little discipline the next day.

I am trying to explain, in simple terms, that everybody can understand how the 21 Day Metabolic Diet works. For this purpose, I have demystified the 7 most important elements for you. These are the 7 pillars that make it so successful. It is not my intention to write a scientific treatise. What I want to do is give you visible images to help you understand the reasons why it is so successful. You will be successful because you have followed the recommendations and understood why!

In the following chapters, I explain in detail the 7 pillars of the 21 Day Metabolic Diet and their relationship to each another. This way, if you wish, you can always refer back to them for any future meal planning.

Basically, you have two ways of doing this:

There is the individual, perhaps biologically and educationally more valuable way. However, this way may be more time consuming. The choice of foods, shopping, and organization all need a lot of planning and preparation. On the other hand, it may be more versatile and more fun.

Or you can choose the easier option, prepared in a kind of "bite-size" way for you but not tailored as individually as the first one. Taking a protein powder and nutritional supplements remains the same and ensures your body receives a sufficient basic supply of micronutrients. Only two meals consist of them, making it less time consuming.

One way is not necessarily better than the other. It is your daily life that will dictate which works better for you. If you no longer enjoy peace and quiet, either in your private life or at work, then at least experience the rapid success of this 21 Day Metabolic Diet without any additional stress.

Should you, however, prefer to find the right way of dealing with your weight issues in a thoughtful and careful way, then take the time to create your own way of eating to correct former bad habits.

➡ And yes – you have tried more or less everything successfully!

➡ And yes – you know best what the outcome was!

➡ And yes – you do not need to repeat any more failures

➡ And wouldn´t it make a nice change to have a good new experience?

➡ This is what this book is about – about a new beginning and a life changing experience!

This is the beauty of the 21 Day Metabolic Diet: you are not supposed to embrace a new ideology. You are not encouraged to try a new miracle diet, let alone buy some mysterious powder or pills. You decide, plan and take your own path. We just offer you the know-how and several options. If you are more conscious afterwards of what you eat, buy better quality food and enjoy it more, then you have accomplished a lot for yourself personally – actually, more than we could expect.

Just enjoy the feeling of doing something good for your body in a healthy, fast and simple manner – no matter which of the two ways you choose.

The principle is based on the following 7 pillars:

1. Effective weight loss due to a sensible balance of energy
2. Lasting success by re-setting your "weight memory"
3. Firmer skin and tissue by maintaining or improving your pH balance
4. Maintaining performance levels by reducing oxidative stress and eliminating toxins
5. Positively impacting the immune system by regulating the intestinal flora
6. Strengthening your body, mind and soul: Omega-3 fatty acids
7. Changes to your "inner self"

Off you go!

Either with the information outlined here or without. I wish you lots of fun and joy with it!

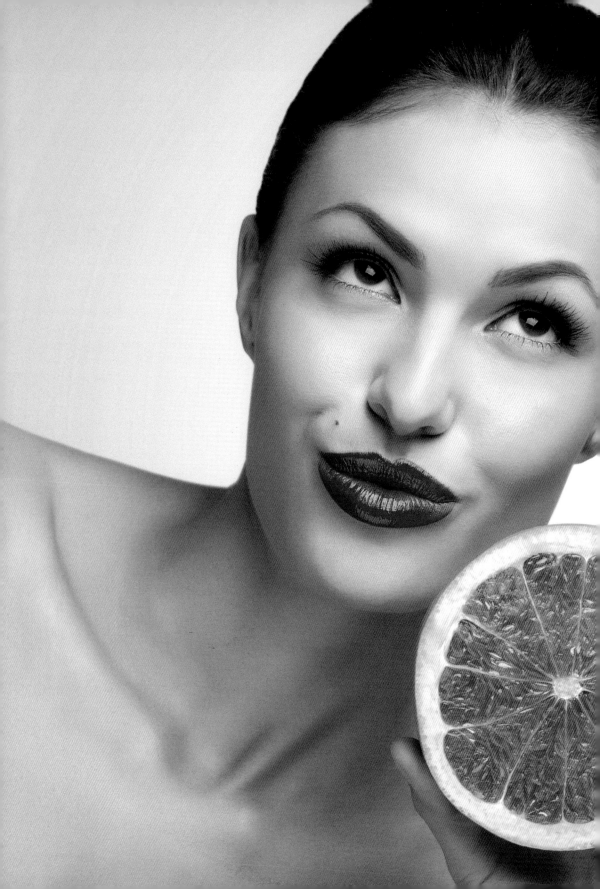

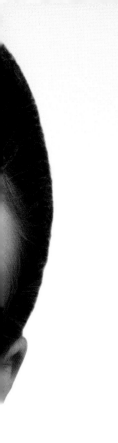

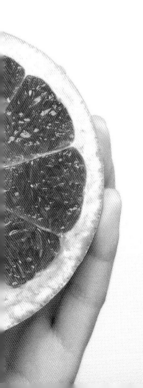

PILLAR 1
Rebalance your metabolism
IN 21 DAYS

EFFECTIVE WEIGHT LOSS
THROUGH CALORIE REDUCTION

1) EFFECTIVE WEIGHT LOSS THROUGH CALORIE REDUCTION

The basics of the 21 Day Metabolic Diet

➡ Three meals per day, in between only water or unsweetened tea

➡ Reduced caloric intake from meals – the rest is provided by the stored body fat

➡ Low fat protein according to the list or suggested recipes

➡ No carbohydrates e.g. bread, potatoes, pasta or rice

➡ No sugar or sweeteners during the 21 days (fruit from the list and only if really necessary)

➡ No fats, oils or butter – avoid oily skin care products

➡ Vegetables, raw food and salad, as much as you like (from the list or the suggested recipes)

➡ No alcohol

It´s easy!

If I want to lose weight I have to provide my body with fewer calories than I burn. This is an inescapable physical law of nature.

> **MEMO:**
>
> *If you want to take your life in a new direction, be sure to pick the right moment.*

Just one thing – over the many thousands of years of evolution it was never intended for us to lose weight on purpose and of our own free will.

For the longest time during our evolution, living conditions were so hostile and difficult that eating was purely for survival at all costs and at all times. Not eating could have easily meant the end for us.

All that mattered was to stay active, walk long distances and find different sources of food. For the longest period of human existence the strategy for survival was to eat everything in sight that was not poisonous.

This also meant that prehistoric man walked about 15 miles a day to find food in order to take in a minimal amount of nourishment for the day. Walking, carrying, foraging, hunting, perhaps even fleeing at some point and, of course, searching for a mate in order to reproduce, that was an everyday chore.

And what did they eat?

Whatever nature had to offer. First of all, this depended on the change of seasons in each part of the world. Furthermore, it depended on the plants and animals prevalent and, finally, on the skills of the individual.

This meant: roots, nuts, bulbs, leaves, flowers, meat, fish, either fresh or dried. In wintertime a little less or even nothing, in summertime a little more and including fruit. Only much later did grains come into the daily diet.

These conditions dictated the entire focus of our bodies, our metabolisms and our survival and it worked very well for a very long time.

And surviving successfully is an advantage, no doubt about that! And these tried and tested advantages have been preserved. This is something our body does automatically – even today.

But let´s be honest: Five meals of fruit and vegetables a day, with bread, pasta, rice, meat and fish and, whenever you feel like it, snacks of chocolate, chips, nuts and ice cream were certainly not the standard fare in prehistoric times.

But it is today:

Most malls are open until 10 pm. Discounters, shopping centers and gas stations are even open around the clock. This means an abundance of food at any time. In addition, we are mostly sitting, starting from daycare to kindergarten and school, apprenticeship or university up until we start working. We move from one place to another mostly by car, bus or metro and, with great pleasure, we spend a large part of our leisure time in front of the computer or other screens. We can easily spend the day lazing on the couch watching numerous programs offered on TV (or DVD) for our entertainment, distraction and supposedly self gratification.

Studies show that an average person in the western hemisphere moves about 600 yards a day!

This means we have a new problem.

Too many calories from food plus too little exercise equals a continually increasing weight!

Of course, this has its consequences: high blood pressure, diabetes, heart attack, stroke, osteoarthritis, dementia and more. This is nothing new and we know it all too well.

The solution is to cut down on calories from food. This way, the body´s reserves will be used up by our daily needs and we will lose weight again. In the prehistoric memory of our body, fewer calories equated to an imminent threat of starvation and would have meant certain death. Of course, our body fights this with all the means it has developed over thousands of years:

➡ A reduction in calories (a lowering of the metabolic rate): any unnecessary waste of energy will be avoided. The less I consume, the longer I can survive. Each cell only works as much as is absolutely necessary, i.e. the blazing flame of our cellular activity turns into smoldering embers.

➡ Muscle loss: if I reduce muscle mass, I can take advantage of additional energy released and cut back future energy consumption (by reducing its main consumer)

➡ A slowing down in the circulation of the blood (poor micro circulation), evidenced by a feeling of cold: the body reduces its operating energy to satisfy its primary energy supply and this way saves additional energy

➡ And as soon as new food is offered: the "yo-yo" effect, quick replenishing of the short-term fat reserves so as to be active as quickly as possible. Afterwards, it increases the long-term reserves (stored body fat) with the understanding: next winter could be even worse. That means: old weight plus X.

This is not new either and many of us know what I am talking about.

Nevertheless, it is important that we are aware of this physiological fact which, up until today, has remained unchanged because these are the tools with which our metabolism has to work. We have no others.

Why is it so difficult then to acknowledge this main pillar of weight reduction and to apply it to everyday life? It is because we find the physical consequences (hunger, feeling cold, physical weakness, discontent, psychological imbalance, restlessness etc.) unpleasant. And what is unpleasant or painful means potential danger! And dangerous things

must be memorized more intensely than pleasant things! This is why we fight things that are unpleasant. We avoid them or try to erase them from our memory banks!

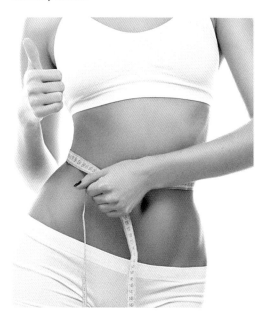

Interestingly enough, these mostly autonomic symptoms (i.e. regulated by the vegetative nervous system and impossible to control) do not develop to such an extent during therapeutic fasting. The body responds to this extreme form of fasting (with no caloric intake except alkaline liquids) with a kind of hunger euphoria. Despite measurable muscle loss, imminent over-acidification and a decrease in the base metabolic rate, we feel extremely agile, ready for action and fit. Even here we see the heritage of evolution: when food is extremely scarce and imminent death by starvation a distinct possibility, a prevailing mood of depression, listlessness and resignation would not be helpful either to our survival or to that of the clan.

For the hunters of the Stone Age, "Get out of the cave and swing that club" had to be their motto in situations such as this.

Besides all the advantages of therapeutic fasting, which are unquestionable, sustainable weight loss is actually not the intended main effect.

So, how can we intentionally bring about a reduction in calories and yet avoid the unpleasant side effects to the body?

By

Pillar 1: choosing the right foods and eating at the right times. (timing)

And

Pillar 2: sensible metabolic regulation by energetic activation (next chapter)

Our nutrition consists of macro and micronutrients. Macronutrients are basic energy building blocks such as carbohydrates, protein and fat. Micronutrients are vitamins, secondary plant compounds, minerals, trace elements and many more. As basic energy builders, they take second stage.

About macronutrients:

Too many carbohydrates and sugar are in the way when you want to lose weight! Carbohydrates consist of simple sugar molecules. The difference between simple sugars and complex carbohydrates can be illustrated best with pearls. When you have a drawer full of single pearls (simple sugars), it is easy to pick them up individually but it is difficult to organize and store them. However, a pearl necklace (complex carbohydrates) is structured, compact, easy to store and, if needed, single pearls can always be cut off.

For example, when you drink a cup of coffee with sugar or when you treat yourself to something sweet, like cake or fruit (yes, fruit also has lots of sugar) you have many pearls at the same time. No matter if they are needed at that time or not: they are there and have to be accommodated. For this purpose the body produces a hormone: insulin.

Figuratively speaking, if our body is a warehouse, insulin is the foreman working in it. When new shipments arrive at the front gate, they will be handled according to: what is needed right away or will get used up right away (e.g. energy for the muscles and, of course, for the brain). What is not immediately required will be put away into small boxes or stored (glycogen) or put away in large boxes and stored (fat). If a truckload of single pearls arrives, it can get hectic. There is a hustle

and bustle of many warehouse workers (insulin) looking for lots of little boxes in which to store the pearls. But since the body does not need so much immediately available energy (single pearls/simple sugars) at that moment, a lot of them have to be stored. During this time all the other work in the warehouse is put aside.

If a shipment of pearl necklaces arrives (e.g. potatoes, pasta, rice, bread) the warehouse foreman can take it easy. First of all, he does not need so many warehouse workers to help him and, second, he has more time to put them away. Whatever is needed for immediate energy can be cut off one after another from a pearl necklace. The others he can store, just as they are.

Once again for clarification: whether the shipment consists of single pearls or pearl necklaces, if it is handled at the front, nothing is being done in the back. There is nobody to open, distribute or resend the pearl necklaces or boxes of pearl necklaces (glycogen or fat) that have been in storage for a long time, let alone use them up. Nothing gets delivered and the storage will not diminish. Just the opposite: it becomes larger and larger and larger!

Weight loss this way? Forget it!

By the way: this analogy is much more memorable than a detailed description of the molecular sequence of the physiological process.

Our brain can only work with simple sugars (glucose). Despite its comparably small percentage in terms of the body's total weight (about 2 %), it uses about 25 % of the entire blood sugar. Hypoglycemia would be a catastrophe for the entire system. Therefore our body has developed a kind of "watchman" to stop this: **Glucagon**.

Glucagon is also a warehouse worker but more in charge of deliveries. Should there be no single pearls (glucose) for the brain available in the foreseeable future, then glucagon comes to its aid. It mobilizes them from the pearl necklaces or boxes of necklaces. Should there come a time when no carbohydrates are supplied but only protein, the warehouse worker, glucagon, goes to work. Translated into real life this means: should there come a time when you only eat protein, more glucagon will be released, however, insulin will only be released in small quantities, to have sugar for the brain. Should this still not be enough, then the "SWAT TEAM" will take over: **Cortisol**. But this means sheer stress and is evidenced by hunger pangs, sweating and shaking.

For our body this means: an equal balance of insulin and glucagon promote a well-balanced metabolism as a result of a well-balanced nutrition. This would come close to our example of "driving straight ahead" at the driving school.

Or put facetiously: should you, over the past few decades, have lived a well-balanced everyday life with a well-balanced diet of the same food with no surprising spectacular occasions or celebrations, then I congratulate you on your ideal weight, yet I feel sorry for you for leading such a boring life!

That is to say our way of life, searching for true fulfillment, is actually designed to be dynamic and not linear. It resembles an "up and down". But this can also get us "out of balance". When it comes to eating, this can quickly lead to becoming overweight. So, what if the warehouse is overflowing? Or in other words: what happens to us "foodies"?

Now we have to be on the look-out for the right choice of food and the right timing.

For us this means: Avoid eating too much sugar and complex carbohydrates. If you do this, less insulin is released and instead glucagon is produced. That´s how it should be!

After carbohydrates we now turn to the proteins mentioned before.

Proteins are the building blocks of life. Whether for the immune system, hormones, enzymes or muscle cells – nothing works without protein. On the other hand, the building blocks for protein are amino acids. Eight of them are essential, i.e. they have to be supplied together with our food. Two others only at certain stages of our lives.

Plants cannot store very much protein which is why the main source of protein in the Western hemisphere comes from animals: meat, poultry, fish, dairy products and eggs. The most well known form of plant protein is soy.

A lack of protein from food leads inevitably to a loss of muscle mass because amino acids are essential for metabolic processes. This is particularly common after a long period of illness or when aging. However, too much protein is harmful as

well, because it cannot be processed and puts a strain on our kidneys as excretory organs. A rule of thumb should be that a palm size piece of meat or poultry provides the necessary quantity of protein (approx. 1.2 oz of pure protein), which is supplied by an equivalent of 5.3 oz of fish or 10.6 oz of Tempeh (a fermented soy product).

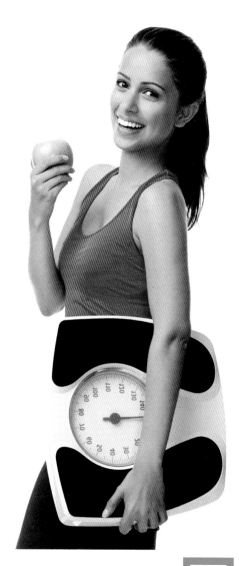

Animal protein often contains more fat as well. Since fat in food is still equated to body fat, many people abstain from protein in favor of carbohydrates. Relevant media campaigns have also played a part in this.

But beware: the absence of fat in food should not be equated to a lack of fat in the body. A latent protein deficiency can often be observed when carrying out such a philosophy to an extreme.

Now let's talk about fat. Basically, there are three different types:

➡ **Saturated fat** – firm at room temperature: e.g. bacon, sausage, pork, full fat quark, butter, whipped cream, cheese etc.

➡ **Monounsaturated fat** – an oily liquid at room temperature: e.g. olive oil, rapeseed oil, almonds, hazelnuts, macadamia nuts etc.

➡ **Polyunsaturated fat** – liquid even when refrigerated: e.g. linseed oil, safflower oil, sunflower oil, tuna, herring, salmon, sardines, walnuts, etc.

Today fats have a frequent and visible purpose as energy reserves ("wobbly fat") and are important building blocks for the cell metabolism. In general they are not as bad as rumoured. They play a major role in the functioning of the metabolism in the brain, the nerves, the blood vessels and also in cell communication. It is all about making the right choices and having the right balance that makes the difference between a healthy and poor diet. For example, monounsaturated and polyunsaturated fatty acids are needed for the optimal functioning of the cell walls. Additional ingredients such as polyphenols (e.g. in olive oil) protect them from oxidation i.e. from becoming rancid and encourage the body to activate the repair mechanisms in the cells.

Nowadays, saturated fats that are consumed in large quantities were not available in the Stone Age. Back then, more lean meat was available instead of pork from pig farms, sausages, cream, cheese and more. However these fats are harmful to the body. Too much of them will cause deposits in the vascular walls, hardened cell membranes, which, in a nutshell, lead to the diseases in civilization that we know all too well.

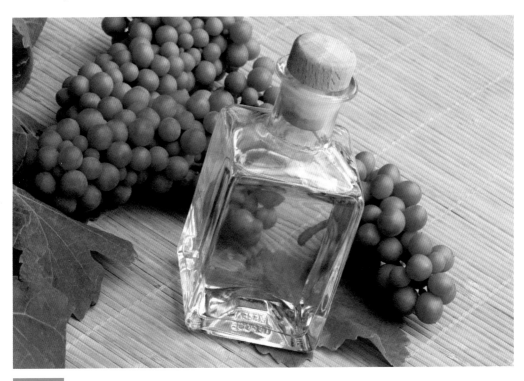

Omega-6 fatty acids and Omega-3 fatty acids are both essential which means they are vitally important and have to be obtained from food. The ratio, however, is no longer correct. Scientists are still debating whether the ratio should be 4:1 or less. Since the ratio is largely decisive for the tissue hormones, an average ratio of 20:1 and more in the Western world, is certainly not health promoting. Tissue hormones (Eicosanoids) have, among other things, an influence on the blood, clotting, inflammatory processes and immune defense. This means refraining from fried foods, ready-made meals, pastries and oils such as sunflower, corn, safflower and soy.

The long-chain Omega-3 fatty acids (the famous fish oil capsules) will be addressed in their own chapter under Pillar 6.

Food for thought:

Every food has its own "biography". Today it is essential to pay close attention to animal husbandry, hidden genetic engineering, organic farming, storage and transportation. The possibilities of increasing profit margins by using chemical and synthetic substances (e.g. to force growth, longer shelf-life, preservation, medication and MSG) have become unmanageable and will eventually be to our cost.

From an ecological and ethical point of view, everyone has to decide how appropriate he thinks industrial livestock farming, animal and food transportation across the country from continent to continent is. This way we certainly reach the most INEXPENSIVE price per pound. However nothing comes as close to your health as your food. Through careful shopping, by not buying cheap goods, you express how much importance you place on your food, your health and the health of your loved ones. Nowadays, nobody is able to judge the quality of food from its appearance and taste. One way out of this dilemma could be, among other things, the regional markets where we, the customer, are still able to buy fresh produce from local farmers.

The easiest way to do Pillar no. 1:

➡ **For breakfast:** Take organic sulfur, antioxidants, vitamins and minerals and fish oil capsules with the protein shake

➡ **For lunch:** Low fat protein with vegetables and salad without oil (see list and recipes)

➡ **For dinner:** Low fat protein with vegetables and salad without oil (see list and recipes). Take organic sulfur and fish oil capsules.

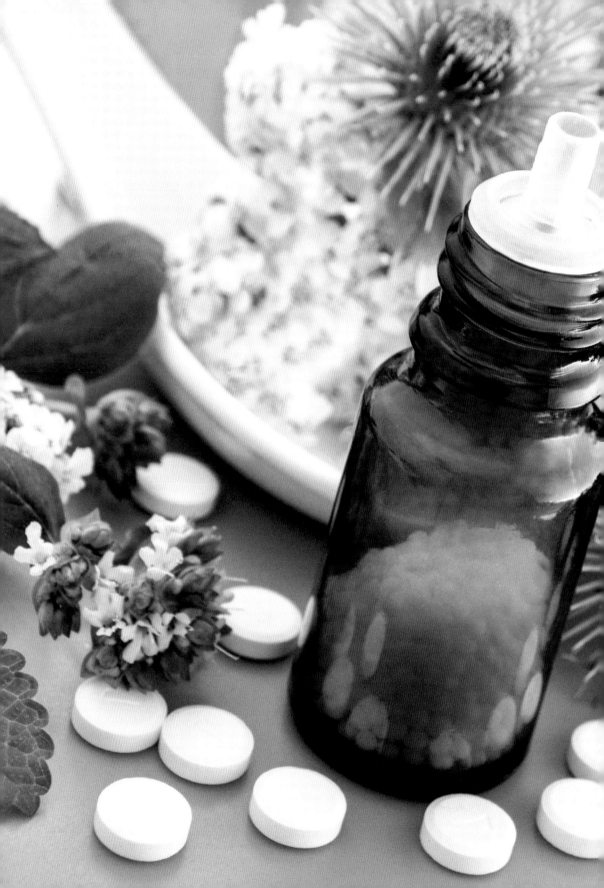

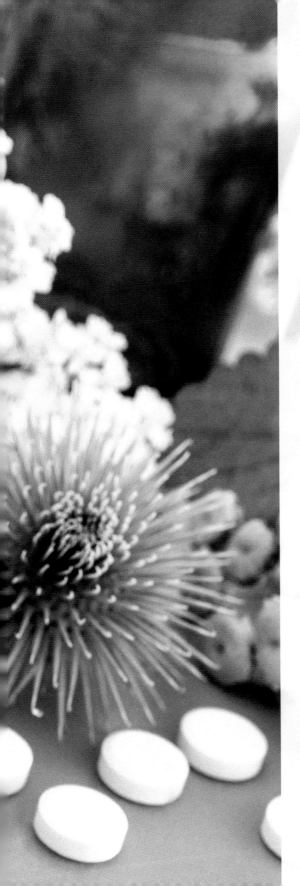

PILLAR 2
Rebalance your metabolism
IN 21 DAYS

ENERGETIC ACTIVATOR –
NO FEELINGS OF HUNGER AND
A NEW WEIGHT MEMORY

2) ENERGETIC ACTIVATOR – NO FEELINGS OF HUNGER AND A NEW WEIGHT MEMORY

The basics during the 21 Day Metabolic Diet

➡ Before meals: morning, midday, evening and before bedtime, take the energetic activator (as globules, drops or other), place under the tongue or allow to dissolve on the roof of the mouth.

➡ Take it at least 20 minutes before brushing your teeth, eating your meals and having coffee

It includes the following:

1. The effect of human chorionic gonadotropin as a chemical messenger for the body

2. The subtle (energetically activated, radionic, homeopathic) use of substances and their effect in particular

First let me talk about human chorionic gonadotropin.

Human chorionic gonadotropin is also known as the pregnancy hormone because it is produced in large amounts especially in the early stages of pregnancy in order to safeguard it.

However, as a matter of fact, it is also detectable in men and women who are not pregnant. It is only produced in larger quantities during pregnancy. In addition to being present in the urine or blood to determine pregnancy, it is also used to monitor the development of certain tumors. In traditional medicine it is used for several therapeutic purposes which are not relevant here.

Research on its effect is still far from over. One thing is for sure, it safeguards the corpus luteum during pregnancy which, in turn, produces progesterone to maintain the pregnancy. Furthermore, in the early stages, it promotes the production of steroid hormones. At this point, I deliberately do not want to go into its inappropriate use in the realm of lifestyle.

This biochemical messenger is of particular interest to us because of the records left by Dr. Albert T.W. Simeons. In his 1954 book, "Pounds and Inches", Simeons documented his observations and conclusions regarding certain effects that, even today, have defied scientific explanation. His hypothesis appears logical, the biological evidence, however, has not been able to be proven (as yet) and for this reason his conclusions have been rejected.

On his numerous journeys and visits to Africa and Asia (as a doctor for the British colonial power) he was able to observe again and again that pregnant women, despite limited food and strenuous physical exertion, were able to keep up their performance and a normal increase in weight. From his point of view, this contradicted the common metabolic theory. He surmised that the answer to this question lay in the hypothalamic-adrenal-pituitary axis. When he evaluated the data of pregnant Indian women, he noticed that they did not experience excessive hunger, despite continuing to work hard with no marked increase in food. Although these women were burning off much higher amounts of energy, they gave birth to healthy babies with no sign of any defects and after pregnancy they quickly regained their former weight.

He assumed a hormonally influenced circuit board, which

1. Maintains the metabolic rate and keeps the flame burning, despite a lack of caloric intake,

2. Maintains muscle mass due to the production of steroids

3. Is able to dissolve real fat deposits from evolutionary related areas (waist, legs, buttocks)

4. Can inhibit feelings of hunger (author's note: probably because of the reduction of leptin resistance when stored fat is dissolved)

5. Is able to re-program our weight memory (set point theory)

These are the effects observed and described by Dr. Simeons! As mentioned above, to date there has been no scientific consensus.

Nevertheless, as a traditional medical doctor who is working in a holistic way, I am extremely cautious when it comes to providing a hormone produced by the body itself that is not actually necessary. Since we have not yet understood all the complex relationships and cannot speculate on many uncertainties, there must be a very viable and nec-

Set point theory

This theory implies that human body weight is genetically/epigenetically programmed and stored and, in the long run does not just succumb to any random influence. Instead it needs to be reset by a coordinating control center (presumably the hypothalamus) to return to its starting point. This initial weight is called the set point weight. It is believed that by overeating for a longer period, the body is able to surpass this initial set point (see Richard Keesey et al.)

essary (therapeutic) reason to justify such a massive invasion of the body´s own hormone system including all known and unknown consequences. From the medical standpoint, an unnecessary hormone treatment must be strictly rejected.

There are more sophisticated ways:

And this brings us to the purely energetic forms of activation, that is to say, radionically or other similar possibilities of subtle activation.

I also cannot give you any new scientific, chemical or physiological evidence. However, using this form of administration, free of any side effects, I see exactly the same changes that I described above!

An analogy:

Imagine from now on you want to admire your living room in a bright orange color. You could go out and buy some orange paint and paint everything orange: the walls, ceilings, floor, couch, chest, TV etc. It is true everything would now be orange, however, it would no longer serve its original purpose. This is a very radical approach with considerable side effects (chemical hormone treatment).

And now imagine you just go and buy some orange light bulbs and, in this way, turn your whole living room orange. You have effectively fulfilled your purpose but the original function of your furniture remains completely unaffected (energetic activation, radionic activation).

This is how you can imagine the energetic influence on your body. There is no material impact on body processes. Only the information of a possible development is introduced to the body. And as a part of its normal physiology, your body can use this information to its advantage by itself and with no external chemical influence!

One thing is clear: we all, whether supporters or opponents of energetic activation, radionic or similar strategies, lack the necessary and comprehensive knowledge in physics, chemistry, biology and physiology to explain, prove or reject how they work. Currently nobody can. Unfortunately, in this regard, there are still too many differences of opinion and I do not wish to take part in this polemic. I shall leave it at that when it comes to proof.

Those who consider it important to pay close attention to effects on the body, mind and soul that go far beyond the purely random, are comfortable with this world of energetic activation.

For those who don´t – without resentment or reproach I recommend you skip the following pages and do not waste your energy or time on things in which you do not believe.

However, please have the control, generosity and tolerance to follow the instructions on how to take our energetic activators (e.g. as globules, radionically activated globules, drops or salt) and simply be curious and watch what happens when you do.

Radionics go back to the American pathologist Dr. Albert Abrams (1863-1924). It is a nonmaterial form of diagnostics and therapy. Under the assumption that each property and action of a substance can be considered as a vibration, a carrier gets electromagnetically activated with the desired information by means of an electrical device. This is when they speak about an activator in the form of globules, salt or an alcohol solution.

In Europe today, the meticulous collection of observations of the German physician Samuel Hahnemann represents the basis of energetic or subtle activation (homeopathy). Based on Hippocrates´ saying: "Like cures like", Hahnemann began to research the effect of different substances on the body, mind and soul.

He did this sometimes by means of questionable experiments on himself, which he documented in great detail. Based on these findings, he manufactured so-called potencies, whereby the original substance was diluted in a certain way in a liquid and then successively diluted and finally agitated.

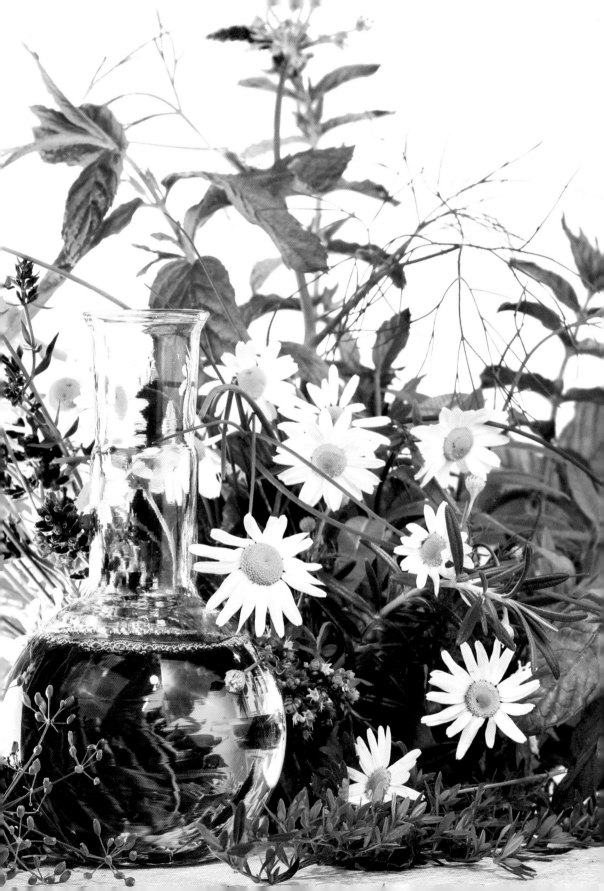

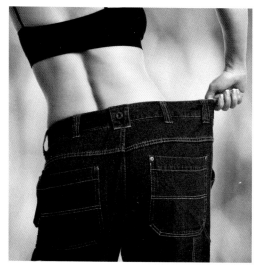

This procedure – as the theory goes – allows the properties of the original substance (also called signatures) to mix with the liquid to a point where the molecules of the original substance are not even traceable, only the information on the properties of the original substance. This way the liquid or sucrose (globules) that has been coated with it can be used therapeutically.

Our energetic activator is intended to work in the same way. The actual information in this messen-

ger substance consists of the mobilization of all strategies to preserve nascent life:

➡ Physical balance in terms of energy supply, even in times of scarcity

➡ Conservation of structures necessary for movement (muscles) to be able to forage, pick or flee

➡ Drawing on unnecessary fat deposits during periods of hunger

➡ Preservation of emotional harmony during difficult times and periods of high caloric consumption

➡ Fast recovery of the body's make-up after birth

The basics of our 21 Day Metabolic Diet Program is:

➡ Taking the energetic activator regularly, 4-5 times per day, with sufficient time between eating, drinking coffee and brushing the teeth (approx. 20-30 minutes)

The easiest way to do Pillar 2:

➡ An experienced therapist who is working in a holistic way will be delighted to help you find this energetic activator as messenger of human chorionic gonadotropin.

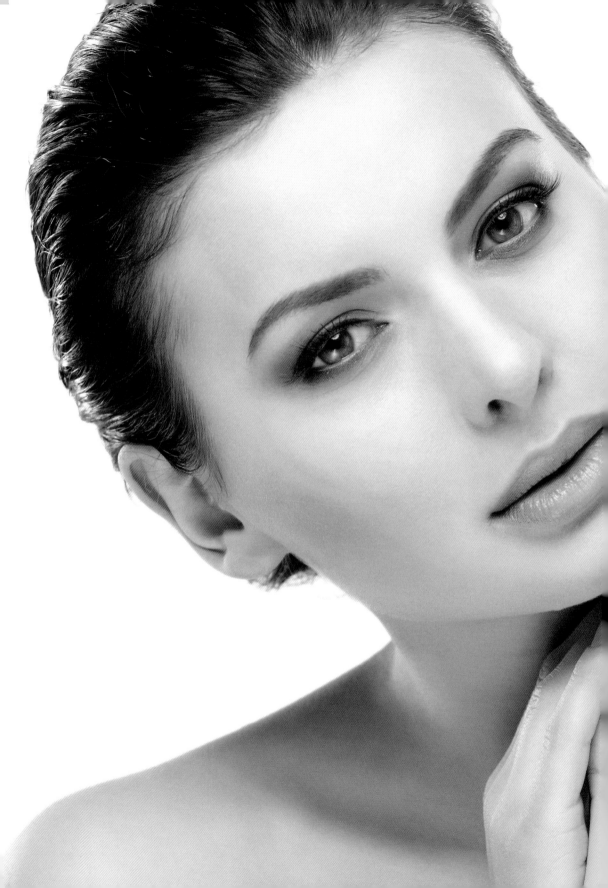

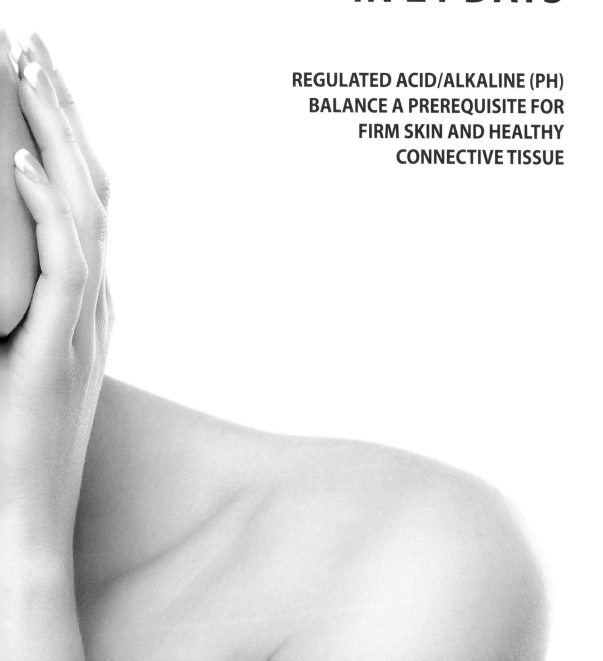

Rebalance your metabolism
IN 21 DAYS

REGULATED ACID/ALKALINE (PH) BALANCE A PREREQUISITE FOR FIRM SKIN AND HEALTHY CONNECTIVE TISSUE

3) REGULATED ACID/ALKALINE (PH) BALANCE A PREREQUISITE FOR FIRM SKIN AND HEALTHY CONNECTIVE TISSUE

The basics during the 21 days

➡ Eat vegetables and salads as alkaline providers of minerals from food (a great variety and a large quantity), if possible, no fruit

➡ Observe the amounts of protein specified

➡ Take alkaline supplements as powder, tea or full baths (optional)

➡ Consciously try to avoid stress in your everyday life to reduce acidification

Still a subject that can cause heated and sometimes polemic discussions is the acid/alkaline (pH) balance of the body and how necessary it is to be aware of it.

The following facts, however, are undisputed:

1. All the metabolic functions of the body's cells can run more or less efficiently. One factor, which has a direct influence is the acid/alkaline balance of the environment of the cell. This acid/alkaline balance can be measured as pH. The lower the value, the more acidic a substance and the higher, the more alkaline. When a substance is neutral, the acid and alkaline values are the same. When this occurs, the pH balance is defined as 7.0. In order to neutralize acids we need what we call "buffers". There are several buffer systems in our body (bicarbonate buffer, hemoglobin buffer, protein buffer, phosphate buffer). If they are depleted the body has to mobilize its remaining reserves, which, among other things, can lead to the bone decalcification of the bones.

MEMO:

Love your life and try everything. Look out for risks and take advantage of any opportunities.

2. At 7.4, the pH of the blood is slightly alkaline. Only two organ systems have a mostly acidic environment: the gastro-intestinal area to kill possible bacteria in the food and to break down the chyme and/or to keep the healthy intestinal bacteria happy. The bladder is the other area that is somewhat acidic, especially in the morning when metabolic waste has to be eliminated (mostly urgently) through the urine.

3. The term "slag" is used in the metallurgical industry and describes the non-metallic, solidified waste from metal smelting, which consists of acid and alkaline oxides (see: Wikipedia). Waste products such as "slag" have never been made visible in the human body let alone been scientifically proven. Nevertheless, the term is often used in reference to the body's metabolic waste. Eliminating naturally produced metabolic waste from the body is called "deslagging". This is precisely the term I would like to use to bring the meaning across in the following chapter!

Many people uphold that "deslagging" of the body is unnecessary. Their argument is: the elimination of acids (visible as acidic urine) and the fact that up until now it is unable to be detected in the tissues shows that the body is capable of neutralizing itself and never needs help from external sources.

However, this is only half the truth because there are situations in which the body´s system of purification fails or is unable to cope effectively. If so, dialysis centers all over the world would be closed right now. In these tragic cases, the kidneys are in a state of renal failure and the body has to be detoxified and deacidified through an external method of waste removal: hemodialysis. Could there be other circumstances that warrant support before reaching such a terminal stage?

I would like to come up with another analogy:

Let´s talk about highway 405 in Los Angeles which, among others, connects the airport and the beaches of Santa Monica with the San Fernando Valley. Over 300,000 cars are using this expressway on a daily basis and traffic jams are the order of the day. However, there are two things that can make it even worse: first of all when an accident or construction work makes the free flow of traffic impossible. And second when, on holidays like Thanksgiving or Christmas, all 3.8 million inhabitants of Los Angeles seem to be trying to reach their destination by car all at the same time. In the first scenario, any "detoxification" has been impeded or made impossible. This happens in the human body as well when the kidneys experience complete renal failure and this is what, in the end makes dialysis necessary. In the second instance, detoxification runs smoothly. However the sudden onslaught of too many cars swamps the roads and causes a backlog. It is simply disastrous when both scenarios happen at once. Can the same thing happen in the body?

Absolutely. Any action of a body cell will only first be made possible through the energy of the cell motor. And this action, which leads to the production of a new substance, is called metabolic process. Simply put, once this process is finished, there are three things that are left: the end product, those elements which were not used, and the exhaust fumes from the motor. These waste products are simply acidic and harmful for the cell itself and its rather alkaline environment. So what should we do with the waste products or "slag" that have accumulated? For one single cell, not a problem: just get rid of it. But when it comes to something as complex as the body, we have developed a special waste disposal system.

"Slag" is transported from one place to another much like the bucket brigade at a fire.

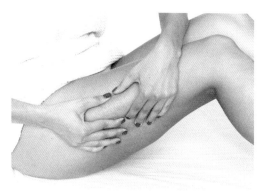

It goes from the cell into the connective tissue with its intracellular matrix (I will explain intracellular matrix later), from the intracellular matrix through the walls of the capillary vessels into the blood and along with the blood into the excreting organs (lung, intestines, kidneys, skin) and, from there, finally to the outside world. (e.g. as exhaled breath, stools, urine or sweat).

The intracellular matrix is a latticework comprised of sugar-protein molecules with numerous ramifications that surround the connective tissue cells.

It is visually similar to a toilet brush. The ends of the bristles are negatively charged and can make a connection with the positively charged acidic waste holding on to it until it can get handed over to the blood. This way the intercellular matrix can be considered as our interim waste storage facility. It is true that the intercellular matrix can be determined chemically, however it is unable to be seen under the electron microscope.

From the perspective of a person with healthy kidneys, a sudden increase in "slag" can only be attributed to a higher metabolic rate. This can occur due to any rigorous demand on the body that goes beyond the normal e.g. illness, stress (physical, intellectual or psychological), extreme sports, poor lifestyle but also from a deliberate reduction in weight. Although desired and initiated on purpose, an increase of cellular breakdown causes the release of more waste.

Now what happens when everything gets too much?

Let's go back to the analogy.

First of all there will be a traffic jam on the expressway. Cars can use the hard shoulder until the traffic comes to a standstill even there.

Going back to the body, the blood as a buffer will bind the increase of acidic "slag" and neutralize it as long as buffer substances in the blood are available. This is only possible up to a certain degree. Physiologically, the body maintains a pH balance of 7.4. If these buffers are exhausted, the result will be another backlog.

The roads that feed into the expressway will get fuller and fuller and finally traffic will come to a standstill there as well.

In the body, the intracellular matrix is used as an additional interim storage facility. Visually this means the bristles of the toilet brush are getting clogged. More and more waste is filling up the intracellular matrix until it becomes overloaded. On the other hand, the intracellular matrix is also the line of communication between the cells. It is like a market place where the latest gossip is heard. How understandable and swift can this conversation be if it is as crowded as Times Square on New Year's Eve before the famous ball drop? Translated to the body, this again means that any metabolic processes have to be carried out under significantly more difficult conditions. The situation can be compared to the cold start-up of a car in winter. There is actually nothing wrong but somehow nothing runs smoothly.

Once the intracellular matrix is overloaded as well, the "slag" backs up as far as the cell. And now it brings about structural damage to the cell and thus to the organ the cell belongs to. This can be avoided, but how?

By introducing more alkaline substances into the body to counterbalance the acidic ones. By increasingly neutralizing these acidic waste products, the threat of a functional disorder or organ damage is contained, despite a large volume of "slag". The detoxifying organs can cope with the extra work and the traffic jam disperses.

This can be done in different ways: First and foremost through diet. Vegetables, salad and fruit work like acid binders in the body, meaning that they are alkaline. Yes, that is correct. Also fruits with their fruit acid can bind other mild acids and in this way have an alkaline effect.

In the following chart you will find a list of assorted foods that are eaten often and their approximate acid load on the body.

Besides you will find the so-called PRAL value (potential renal acid load for 3.5oz of the respective food, indicated in meq (physical and chemical milli-equivalents). High minus values mean very alkaline, high plus values mean very acid.

Modified according to Remar and Manz, Journal of the American Dietetic Association 1995; 95:791-797).

Acid

Cereals

Cornflakes	6.00
Egg pasta	6.40
Oatmeal	10.70
Parboiled rice, cooked	1.70
Rice, polished, raw	4.60
Rice, unpolished, raw	12.50
Rye bread	4.10
Rye crispbread	3.30
Rye –wheat bread (50 % rye)	4.00
Whole rye flour	5.90
Spaghetti	6.50
Wholemeal spaghetti	7.30
White bread	3.70
Wheat bread	1.80
Wheat flour	6.90
Wheat-rye bread (50 % wheat)	3.80
Wholewheat flour	8.20

Pulses

Peas	1.20
Lentils, green and brown, dried	3.50

Alkaline

Vegetables

Cauliflower	-0.4
Broccoli	-1.2
Belgian endives	-2.0
Iceberg Salad	-1.6
Cucumbers	-0.8
Carrots, baby	-4.9
Lettuce (average 4 varieties)	-2.5
Leeks	-1.8
Mushrooms	-1.4
Garden radish	-3.7
Asparragus	-0.4
Spinach	-14
Tomatoes	-3.1
Zucchini	-4.6
Onions	-1.5

Pulses

Beans, green	-3.1

Acid

Fruit, nuts and fruit juices

Peanuts, untreated	8.3
Walnuts	6.8

Beverages

Coca-Cola	0.4

Fats and oils

Olive oils, sunfloweroil	0.0
Butter	0.6

Fish

Herring	7.0
Codfilet	7.1
Haddock	6.8

Alkaline

Fruit, nuts and fruit juices

Apples, 15 varieties, with peel, average	-2.2
Apple juice, unsweetened	-2.2
Apricots	-4.8
Bananas	-5.5
Strawberries	-2.2
Grapefruit juice, unsweetened	-1.0
Hazelnuts	-2.8
Cherries	-3.6
Kiwi	-4.1
Oranges	-2.7
Orange juice, unsweetened	-2.9
Peaches	-2.4
Raisins	-21.0
Black currants	-6.5
Water melon	-1.9
Lemon juice	-2.5

Beverages

Beer, Pilsener	-0.2
Coffee, steeped 5 minutes	-1.4
Hot chocolate, made from skim milk (3.5 %)	-0.4
Mineral water, sparkling	-1.8
Mineral water, still	-0.1
Red wine	-2.4
Tea, Indian, steeped	-0.3
Tomato juice	-2.8
White wine	-1.2

Fats and oils

Margarine	-0.5

Fish

Acid

Meat and cold cuts

Corned beef, can	13.2
Frankfurter	6.7
Luncheon meats, can	10.2
Chicken	8.7
Veal	9.0
Liversausage	10.6
Beef, lean	7.8
Rumpsteak, lean or fat	8.8
Salami	11.6
Pork, lean	7.9
Turkey	9.9

Milk, dairy products

Buttermilk	0.5
Camembert	14.6
Cheddar, reduced fat	26.4
Egg whites	1.1
Fruit yogurt, full fat	1,2
Gouda	18.6
Hard cheese, average 4 varieties	19.2
Egg	8.2
Cottage cheese, full fat	8.7
Evaporated milk	1.1
Icecream, vanilla	0.6
Yogurt, natural, full fat	1,5
Parmesan	34.2
Quark	11,1
Sour cream	1.2
Processed cheese	28.7
Full milk, pasteurized and homogenized	0.7
Soft cheese, full fat	4.3

Sugar, preserves and sweets

Milk chocolate	2.4
Pound cake	3.7

Alkaline

Meat and cold cuts

Milk, dairy products

Sugar, preserves and sweets

Honey	-0.3

There are numerous other charts today which may be more accurate. I personally like this chart very much and I think for our purposes it is absolutely fine.

Of course you can work with alkaline teas or alkaline powders, tablets or capsules, especially if you feel a little uncomfortable at the beginning of the diet.

Alkaline baths can take the edge off these unpleasant symptoms and they can also help to improve your skin, which is supposedly achieved by deacidifying the body through the skin. In the medical field, they have a lot of success with alkaline intravenous drips. This, however, should be left to experienced physicians, alternative practitioners and therapists and only after a relevant diagnosis.

In reference to weight reduction through the 21 Day Metabolic Diet, the basics for the acid/alkaline (pH) balance is as follows:

➡ Do not exceed the required quantities

➡ From the selection of vegetables and salads, you may wish to be as versatile as possible and choose mostly alkaline varieties

➡ You may wish to add alkalizing products (teas, powders, alkaline baths)

➡ Try to avoid overwhelming daily chores

The easiest way to do Pillar 3:

➡ **Morning:** Protein drink with alkalizing nutritional and mineral supplement (source see p. 154)

➡ **Midday:** In addition to the protein, eat plenty vegetables from the list or recipes

➡ **Evening:** In addition to the protein, eat plenty vegetables from the list or recipes

➡ Accompanied by alkaline teas, ginger tea and sometimes an alkaline bath

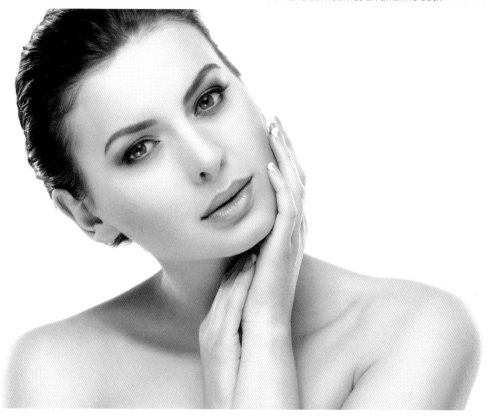

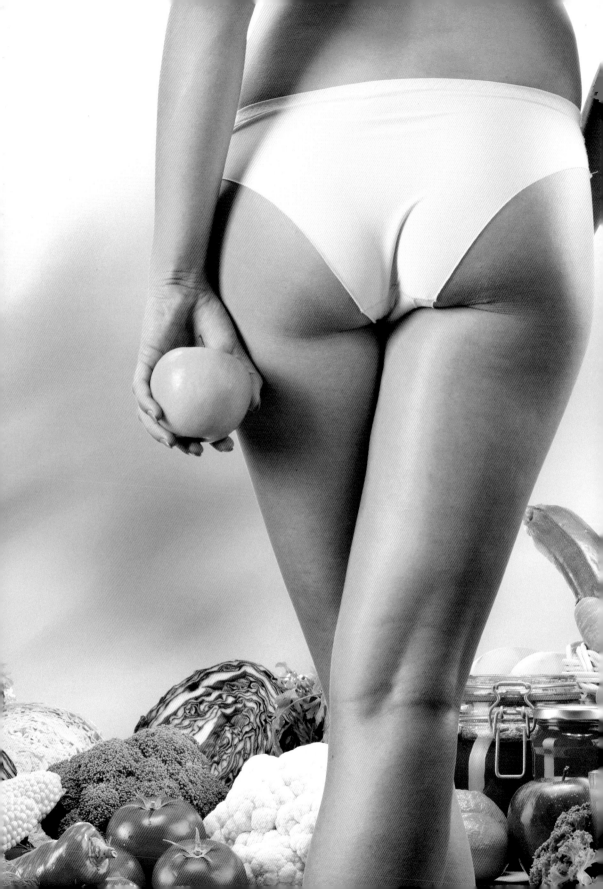

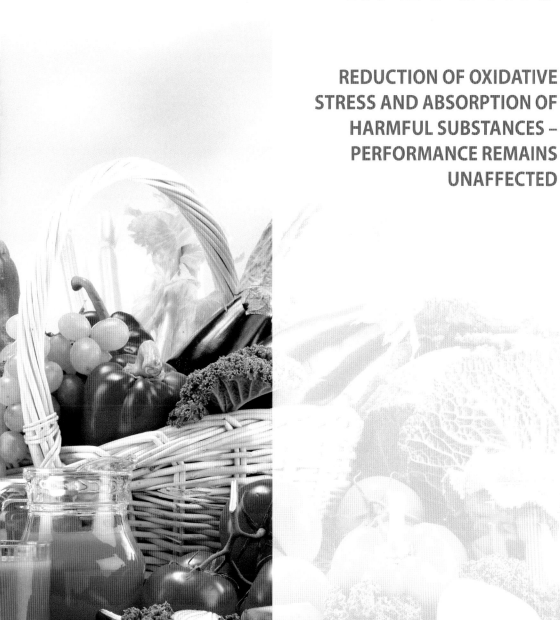

IN 21 DAYS

REDUCTION OF OXIDATIVE STRESS AND ABSORPTION OF HARMFUL SUBSTANCES – PERFORMANCE REMAINS UNAFFECTED

4) REDUCTION OF OXIDATIVE STRESS AND ABSORPTION OF HARMFUL SUBSTANCES – PERFORMANCE REMAINS UNAFFECTED

The basics during the 21 days:

➡ Provide your body with nutrients from vegetables, raw food and salads (see list and recipes)

➡ Due to an increase in the amount of free radicals and the need to eliminate them, give your body micronutrients and antioxidants from nutritional supplements

➡ Take high quality detoxifying supplements and binders such as organic sulfur (MSM) and chlorella

➡ Supplement with Omega-3 fatty acids (to improve the function of the wall of the cell)

With every breath we take, we burn energy and produce metabolic waste. A part of these end products is called free radicals: unstable molecules that are constantly looking for free electrons. They steal these electrons from other molecules and thus are able to damage the structures they affect.

The sum of all these free radicals is called oxidative stress which is a result of the normal metabolic processes in our body. If there is not much going on, there will be less oxidative stress. If there is a lot going on, there will be much more. This is why any physical, cognitive or emotional strain will cause oxidative stress. Even a metabolic rebalancing of the body, such as the 21 Day Metabolic Diet which is done deliberately, will produce metabolic waste and thus more oxidative stress. This metabolic waste must be eliminated as it is harmful for the cells, every cell. Cellular damage becomes visible and noticeable by premature aging and disease which our modern society does not accept as unavoidable anymore. However, opinions are divided when it comes to ways of combating such processes.

Since cosmetic surgery is on the rise, I think this confirms the fact that plenty of sleep, drinking a lot of pure water and getting lots of fresh air are N O T enough for a radiant appearance and feeling of vitality.

Apart from the body´s own "slag" or waste products, we are faced with daily toxic challenges from the environment, some of which cannot be avoided. This puts an increased strain on the body.

These might be heavy metals (e.g. lead, cadmium, mercury), light metals (e.g. aluminum), chemical solvents, petrochemicals, medicinal residue, wood preservatives, hair dye, contamination of foodstuffs, pesticides and biotoxins (toxins from bacteria, viruses and fungi) amongst many others. They all have to be detected, neutralized and eliminated by the body. This will happen in different ways in our body. Sometimes during this process more free radicals can may be produced and this will represent a serious problem and challenge to the body.

Body structures that must be especially protected are the mitochondria (the "power plant" of the cell), DNA (the genetic make-up of the cell), fatty acids (which are especially susceptible to oxidation and destruction), proteins (amino acids which are necessary for the absorption of toxins and other cell structures of the blood vessels and nerves).

Our body uses a variety of antioxidants in order to dispose of free radicals. The body is capable of producing some of them itself (endogenous antioxidants), such as glutathione, ceruloplasmin, albumin, ubiquinone and many more.

Other exogenous antioxidants must be supplied by Vitamin C, Vitamin E, zinc, manganese, copper, selenium, beta carotene, potassium and OPCs

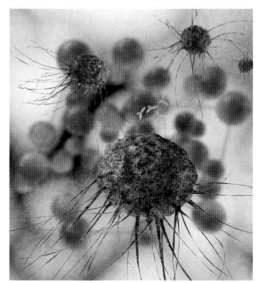

(oligomeric proanthocyanidins also called grape seed extract) and many others. We can provide our body with them by eating food such as vegetables, salad, herbs, seeds and fruit as well as plant oils, soy, tea, coffee, eggs and even red wine. However this is a matter of balance.

Substances that the metabolism needs as catalysts for the detoxification and elimination of waste are called micronutrients. This is not a scientifically defined term. It rather refers to active ingredients which keep us healthy or help us to become healthy again. Actually what is meant is vitamins, minerals, trace elements, secondary plant compounds as well as antioxidants. Their common denominator is that they are not sources of energy. Amino acids and fatty acids are often included in amongst them however they can act as both building blocks and energy for the body. It was, in effect, anthropological research that helped medicine to trace these substances, in particular, by observing and comparing different population groups: their diet, environment, habits, illnesses and their traditional healing methods.

A dissertation on all these active ingredients is beyond the scope of this book. However I would like to address a few of them.

Sulfur

Sulfur is a vitally important mineral playing a huge role in the metabolism of protein and the elimination of waste products. Sulfur is an important component of the connective tissue, the bones, the skin and the hair. The endogenous (body´s own) antioxidants taurine and glutathione can only be produced when sulfur is present.

Heavy metals, chemical solvents and other toxins like to attach themselves to molecules of the cell membrane that should actually be occupied by sulfur. In order to remove cell-bound toxins the body has to be given a high dose of organic sulfur (methylsulphonylmethane, MSM). This is why MSM is a potent detoxifying agent, which is also excellent for dental and gum issues. Now the toxins released have to be eliminated. This requires a binder which, in turn, is used by sulfur groups as the binding molecule. Chlorella algae and also goat whey (with its sulfur-containing amino acids) are especially suitable for this purpose.

Secondary plant compounds

Among the different secondary plant compounds, flavonoids have been recognized since 1930, thanks to Nobel Laureate Albert von Szent-Györgyi Nagyrápolt. Their omnipresence in plants and their mainly antioxidant effect make them extremely valuable to us. Their special effects on our body are as multifaceted as the group itself.

The properties that have been verified and that are most important for us are their anti-allergic, anti-inflammatory, anti-viral, anti-microbial and anti-carcinogenic effects.

Representatives are: lutein (available in dark green leafy vegetables such as kale and spinach for eye protection), lycopene (in tomatoes, for their positive effects on cardio-vascular diseases and cancer), quercetin (e.g. in apples, broccoli, sea buckthorn, cranberries for its anti-carcinogenic effect), and hesperidin (e.g. from citrus fruits for its effect on the lymphatic system and blood circulation. It can also lower cholesterol).

There are two polyphenols from the whole grape that are generally recognized and highly effective: OPCs (Oligomeric proanthocyanidins, in the grape seed) and resveratrol (in the grape skin). OPCs have an incredible antioxidative effect and are especially beneficial for the skin, eyes, immune system and hormone balance. Studies show that resveratrol has a positive effect particularly on arteriosclerosis, Alzheimer and autoimmune diseases. OPCs demonstrate cancer preventing properties as well.

Minerals and trace elements

These are calcium, magnesium, zinc, iodine, copper, manganese, molybdenum, selenium etc.

Magnesium is often described as "the salt of inner peace". It plays a part in over 300 enzymatic reactions and is needed in every metabolic process requiring energy. 95 % of these occur within the cell e.g. in the bones, the heart and skeletal muscles, in the brain, the kidneys, the liver as well as the red blood cells. It reduces the release of stress hormones and is a natural regulator for hyper excitability. In reference to trace elements, I would like to mention zinc and selenium as an example. As a co-enzyme, zinc plays a part in over 300 enzymatic reactions. It participates in the production of enzymes and hormones, the building of DNA, elimination of heavy metals, immune response and many more. Amongst other things, nuts are a good source of zinc. Selenium strengthens the immune system and has an anti-carcinogenic effect (i.e. prevents cancer). In particular, selenium has a positive effect on the detoxification capability of the liver. It protects the eyes from cataracts, ensures a healthy thyroid and protects from degenerative nerve diseases.

Vitamins and Vitaminoids

While it is true that the science concerning the effects of vitamins on our bodies has been fairly comprehensive, it still, however, has a long way to go. The list of positive effects on our lives in terms of health, vitality and wellbeing is too long to find enough room here. However, let me mention the antioxidative effect of Vitamin C and Vitamin E which help us overcome:

➡ Acute and chronic infections

➡ Disorders of the lipid metabolism

➡ Allergies

➡ Toxic loads

➡ Smoking

➡ Stress

➡ Coronary diseases and hypertension

➡ Tumors

➡ Any kind of debility and immune deficiency, and many others

It is already well known to us that we can provide our body with these vitamins by eating vegetables (e.g. kale, white and red cabbage, spinach, broccoli), and fruits (e.g. Billy goat plum, acerola cherry, rosehip, kiwi, citrus fruits). Nevertheless, the amount provided does not always appear adequate.

Vitamin D (Cholecalciferol) has a bone-supporting, cell-maintaining and life-prolonging effect. It has been known for a long time as a prevention and therapy for bone decalcification. However, only recently has it been found that hormone-like effects also keep our body healthy. A lack of Vitamin D seems to be a risk factor not just for osteoporosis but also for allergies, asthma, autoimmune diseases, infectious diseases, dementia, cancer and sterility. The body´s own Vitamin D production in the skin by means of sunlight no longer appears adequate in this day and age.

The B-Vitamins are a vitamin group that acts as early stages of coenzymes. They are available in animal and plant-based foods (except Vitamin B 12 which only occurs in animals) such as, for example, fish, dairy products, liver products, spinach, broccoli and kale. Their role in our body is very diverse. Due to the fact that some of the B Vitamins today are classified as vitamin-like substances, their numbering is not consecutive. This includes choline (before it used to be called Vitamin B4) and folic acid (indicated as Vitamin B11 or Vitamin M). Besides their hematopoietic, nerve protecting and anti-oxidative effects, the entire amino acid metabolism depends on the B Vitamins.

Other vitamin-like substances are L-Carnitine and Ubiquinone (Q 10). L-Carnitine is indispensible for the mitochondria (the power plants of the cells): it liberates the mitochondria from free radicals, protects the membranes, provides them with nutrients and releases energy. Cell vitality without L-Carnitine is simply not possible. Since adults can produce it themselves, it is called a vitaminoid. Just like Ubiquinone (Q10): it takes center stage when it comes to energy production within the mitochondria and can be found in every cell. This alone shows how important this substance is for the body. The importance of Omega-3 fatty acids as a part of the nutritional substances recommended by us will be discussed separately in Pillar 6.

If you have already done something to detoxify your body, that is excellent. Keep it up! But is it enough? It has been proven that the amount of nutrients in our food has decreased. The reasons for this are many and would deserve their own chapter. At the same time, the needs of our bodies seem to have increased due to our modern lifestyle. Nutritional supplements can be a solution.

And what happens during the 21 Day Metabolic Diet? Think about your own home: dusting daily is easy and does not take long because it is just the dust from yesterday to today. However, a complete spring clean of all the rooms, the cellar and the attic kicks up a lot more dirt. The 21 Day Metabolic Diet is such a complete spring clean!

A metabolic rebalance such as this releases many more toxins and free radicals that must be intercepted. This is why we should focus our attention on defense and its tools!

Or, to put it more graphically, imagine at a stadium after a football game all the men's room toilet doors are opened at the same time: what a smell, what a mess!

Now this will call for a thorough cleaning and airing out!

For our 21 Day Metabolic Diet this means:

➡ Receiving enough exogenous nutrients through vegetables, raw food, spices and salads and, in the stabilization phase, also through fruit and oils

➡ Supplementation with high quality nutritional supplements and teas

➡ Supplementation with organic sulfur, perhaps even chlorella or goat whey to flush out toxins, if well tolerated

➡ A daily dose of Omega-3 fatty acids to bind the toxins

Please bear in mind: research has, of course, identified several individual substances that are assumed to have a positive effect on our body and, naturally, these can be manufactured synthetically. The question as to whether it is not the entire package of nutrients in our food that is responsible for our health remains open. Science always pays attention to the health promoting effects of our food and its entire cocktail of ingredients, not just one molecule! That is to say: the best thing is the careful preparation of organic food as a whole. And please do always give priority to nutrients derived from natural sources. They store the entire composition of regenerating nutrients and not just a tiny part.

An opera at the Metropolitan Opera House becomes an unforgettable experience because of the whole orchestra, not just the first clarinet (although he is the one playing the melody).

The easiest way to do Pillar 4:

➡ **Morning:** Take organic sulfur, antioxidants, vitamins and minerals and fish oil capsules with the triple protein shake.

➡ **Midday:** Meal according to the list or recipes, with lots of fresh vegetables and salad

➡ **Evening:** Meal according to the list or recipes, with lots of fresh vegetables and salad, together with organic sulfur and fish oil capsules.

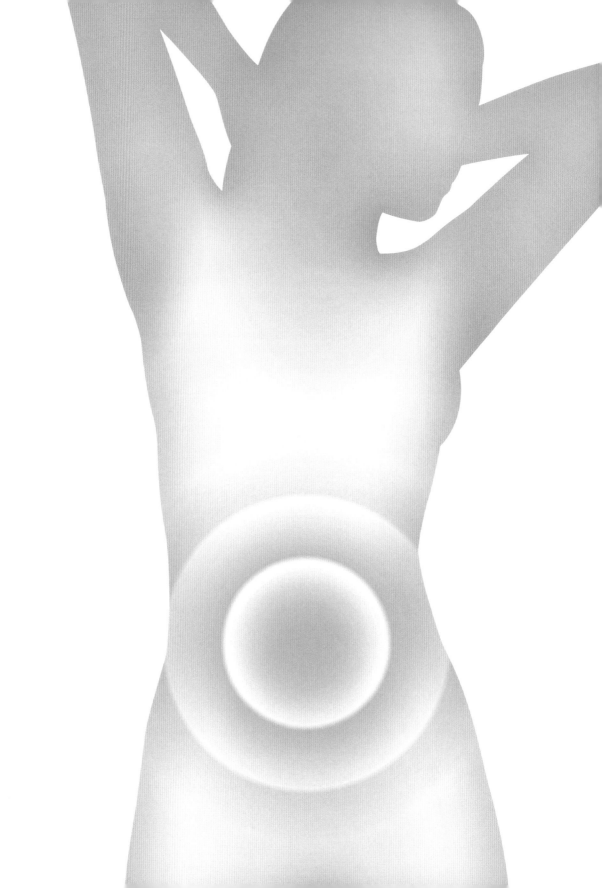

Rebalance your metabolism
IN 21 DAYS

A HEALTHY INTESTINAL FLORA IMPROVED IMMUNE SYSTEM AND OPTIMAL SUPPORT FROM NUTRIENTS

5) A HEALTHY INTESTINAL FLORA IMPROVED IMMUNE SYSTEM AND OPTIMAL SUPPORT FROM NUTRIENTS

The basics of the 21 Day Metabolic Diet:

➡ Cooked and sautéed foods are easier than raw food and salads for the intestines to digest

➡ Additional probiotics from lactobacilli and the bifidobacterium group.

➡ Prebiotic support through fiber-rich vegetables like Belgian endives, salsify and more.

"Together we are strong!"

This is how our body´s motto has to be understood in terms of working closely with the numerous microorganisms inside it.

Our nose and throat, our bronchial and intestinal area, all these places are populated by microscopically small cohabitants. For the 21 Day Metabolic Diet, we only need to interest ourselves in the large and small intestines. Their outer mucous membranes provide the ideal habitat for a variety of favorable and unfavorable microorganisms.

The large and small intestines have a surface which is folded several times. If we were to completely unfold this "carpet" (including even the microscopically small wrinkles, the so-called micro villi) their surface area would be over 20,000 sq ft which is almost as large as half a football field. And there are approximately 100 trillion bacteria from about 500 different bacterial strains meaning we have almost 100 times more microorganisms than we have body cells. These numbers are huge and hard to comprehend.

But let us try: Imagine one volume of a dictionary. (Yes, you are right. I am from the pre-Wikipedia

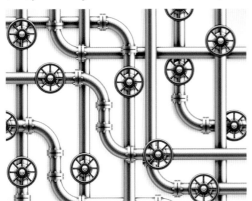

era). 200 characters per line, 50 lines per page and 100 pages will make it half an inch thick. If now one volume is lined up next to another in a row as long as from New York to Miami, the amount of printed characters in all those volumes would correspond to the amount of bacteria in our intestines. These bacteria weigh all together about 2 pounds. Approximately 2 thirds of all the body's immune cells are found around the intestines (in the connective tissue and the surrounding lymphatic system). This is why we often call the intestines the center of the immune memory.

How is our intestinal flora created?

The first bacterial colonization begins at birth when mostly lactobacilli and bifidobacteria are transferred from the vaginal canal of the mother to the newborn. Unfortunately, the first problems can arise with baby food. Putrefactive bacteria can feed on a part of the fiber in baby food causing bloating and colic-type intestinal cramping. This lowers the natural acidity of the intestines which is not as beneficial for the good intestinal bacteria. The normal development of the immune system still needs some time. If at this time there are no antibodies from breast milk (because breast feeding is impossible or undesired) then the first contact with pathogenic bacteria can lead to serious diseases and later to a damaged immune system with food intolerances, allergies or atopic dermatitis.

The possibility or impossibility to breast feed, or the voluntary or involuntary decision to use baby formula, influences the further development of our intestinal flora and thus our entire future.

The bacterial colonization of the stomach, the intestines and the colon will only be completed in the second year. This is when the stomach has very little bacteria and the small intestine has lactobacilli and enterococci. The higher acidity in the small intestine is caused by the fermentation of carbohydrates through lactobacilli and serves as a protective barrier. However the thickest layer of bacteria can be found in the colon. These bacteria in the colon cannot migrate upwards to the small intestine due to its higher acidity. Therefore the colon is colonized by bifidobacteria, eubacteria, bacteroids and approximately 1 % of escherichia coli and enterococci. If the amount of the latter increases, dysbiosis, which is an unfavorable process of putrefaction, will start in the intestines: the food is not digested and broken down properly so the intestines are unable to complete other functions as they should.

The basic purpose of our intestinal flora is:

➡ Optimal breakdown of chyme, thus supporting digestion for the best use of nutrients

➡ Defense against harmful organisms (including parasites, fungi and viruses) and their toxic waste products by developing a continuous layer of bacteria.

➡ Development and permanent control of a healthy immunocompetence

➡ Supply of vitamins from bacterial metabolic activity (thiamine, Vitamin B2, B12, Vitamin K)

➡ Energy supply to the intestinal epithelial layer and increase in bowel movement towards the rectum through butyric acid (made from intestinal bacteria)

➡ Detoxification

None of these functions can be carried out properly if the intestinal flora is compromised. It is understood and has been known for a long time that this causes an increase in intestinal problems (e.g. bloating, constipation, diarrhea) and diseases (e.g. infections, intestinal inflammations, rheumatic diseases, cancer).

Throughout our entire life our daily behavior influences our intestinal flora. Everything we ingest, we surround ourselves with, and somehow become influenced by, has a positive or negative effect on our intestinal flora: Eating, drinking, smoking, medication, pollutants, radiation but also infections, injuries, chronic diseases, stress, psychological strain and emotional distress.

In such cases the following approach would be of benefit:

1) If possible, avoid any further negative influences

2) Improve the intestinal flora by taking probiotics and prebiotics. This is called symbiotic control.

Probiotics are "good" live bacteria (predominantly lactobacilli, bifidobacteria, but also Escherichia coli strains), whose role, much like that of a teacher, is to show the intestinal bacteria how to function properly.

Prebiotics are non-digestible food ingredients which, however, specifically stimulate certain types of bacteria in the intestines. For the most part these are di-, oligo- and polysaccharides such as, for example, inulin, lactulose, oligofructose and many others.

The decision to rebalance your metabolism in 21 days by following our recommendations creates a new challenge for your intestines and their cohabitants.

Since this is a physiological change, which is useful for life, your intestines will grow with this task. Trust your body! Known for years already and proven time and time again, this rebalancing has long-term health benefits. Your body´s ability to react to its environment will significantly improve.

In terms of our 21 Day Metabolic Diet this means:

Food should be easy to digest. If you have a delicate digestive system, as a rule, vegetables are recommended because everything that is cooked, sautéed or blanched can be broken down more easily by the body than raw food or salads. Please note that short cooking times will prevent valuable nutrients from being destroyed. Leafy salads, tomatoes and sprouts are easily digestible. Belgian endives, salsify and Jerusalem artichokes are rich in natural prebiotics.

MEMO:

If I lower my expectations to a minimum, life will turn into a series of surprises.

Take a tour of discovery! Be a pioneer again, ready to take some risks! Get curious and try out new things: there are far more vegetables available than you have ever had on your menu up until now.

Fats should be used sparingly and never overheated (this happens with frying and repeat heating). This could cause an unfavorable flow of bile and the resultant metabolic components could cause diarrhea. During the production of hydro-

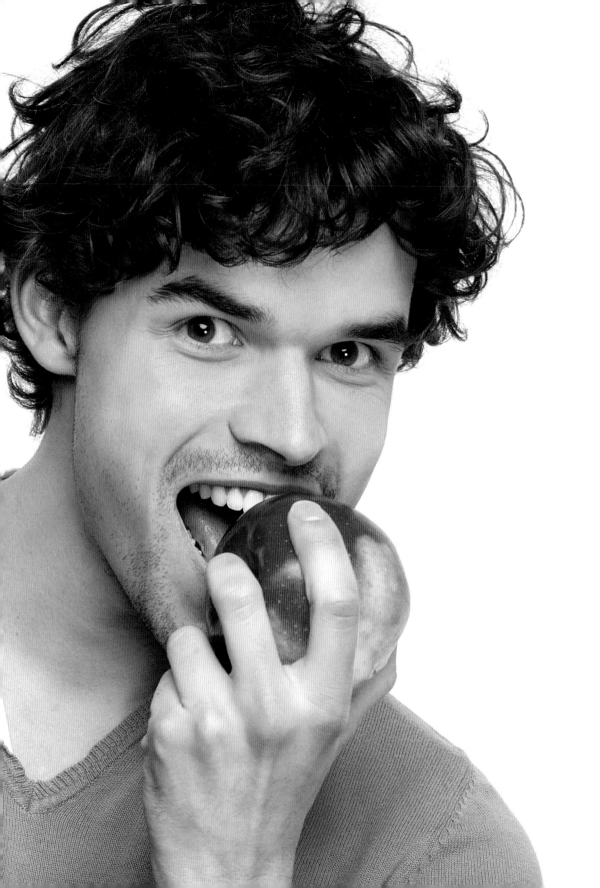

genated fats, the so-called "trans fats" increasingly occur and these are harmful to your health. So then, eat considerably fewer French fries, cookies and potato chips and less processed food, fast food and margarine.

Plant oils used for vegetables and salads are good and important. However, for frying meat, they are somewhat unsuitable due to their low smoke point and the resultant molecular change. (See Pillar 6 for Cis and Trans explanation)

As for meat, the lighter, leaner and more tender varieties such as veal, poultry and turkey are preferable. Dark meat such as beef, game and mutton should be chewed especially well so as not to allow any room for putrefactive bacteria. Of course, non oily fish is also recommended. Take your time when frying or sautéing. It is neither good nor necessary to eat grilled or breaded meat all the time.

Okay, I agree, for many people that's a massive change to their everyday life!

And yes, a change to your everyday life requires greater effort!

And yes, one or two of these changes will be difficult to incorporate into your everyday life because they are new and unusual!

But don't you think it is exciting to leave an old habit behind and try something new on your way to success?

Regarding your choice of probiotics, you should rely on the advice of an experienced physician. In the meantime, there is such a huge variety on the market that you can hardly see the forest for the trees. Although it is highly unlikely that you could harm yourself by choosing an inappropriate product, your investment should be as good as it can be. So you had better ask the expert. If in doubt, a biological, natural yoghurt is a good start after the 21 Day Metabolic Diet.

The easiest way to do Pillar 5:

➡ **Morning:** Include pro- and prebiotics in your protein shake or get them from other recommended sources.

➡ **Midday and evening:** The choice and preparation of both of your individual meals, following the above mentioned explanations and recipes, forms the basis for a favorable development of the intestinal flora. Your intestines will adapt to your new metabolic condition after the 21 Day Metabolic Diet, although it may be unfamiliar at first.

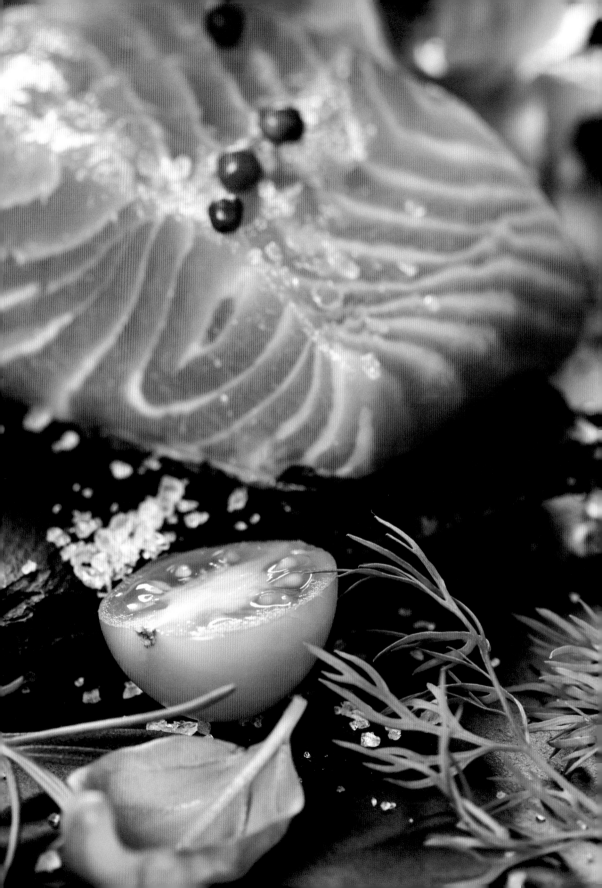

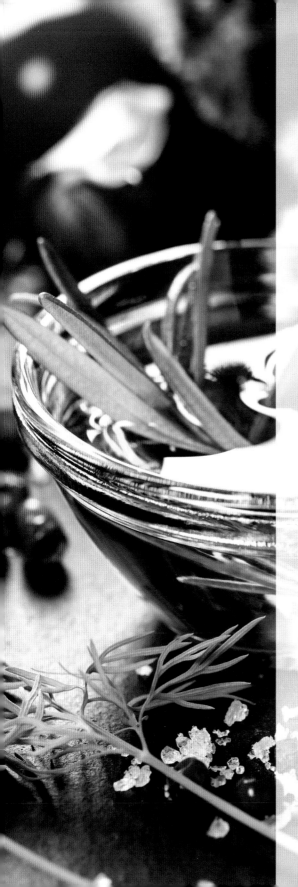

PILLAR 6
Rebalance your metabolism
IN 21 DAYS

STRENGTHENING OF BODY, MIND AND SOUL – OMEGA-3 FATTY ACIDS

6) STRENGTHENING OF BODY, MIND AND SOUL – OMEGA-3 FATTY ACIDS

The basics of the 21 Day Metabolic Diet

➡ Steamed coldwater fish from unpolluted, clean fishing grounds

➡ Fish or krill oil capsules of high quality, pollution free manufacture

➡ High quality antioxidants, micronutrients and secondary plant compounds from vegetables, raw food and salads to preserve the valuable Omega-3 fatty acids

Now we are getting into chemistry: but don´t worry too much!

It´s all about Omega-3 fatty acids. Why?

Because historical research shows that cardio-vascular diseases among the Inuit in Greenland are conspicuously rare, despite their very fatty diet, researchers began to search for the reason for this and discovered Omega-3 fatty acids.

What are fatty acids?

Fatty acids are long, linear hydrocarbon chains with a so-called carboxyl group at their ends.

Fats are a combination of glycerine and fatty acids.

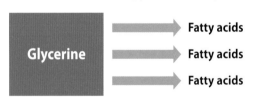

If all three binding sites of the glycerine are occupied, we speak of triglycerides, which are almost exclusively contained in our dietary fats.

Fatty acids can either be (as described before) saturated, monounsaturated or polyunsaturated fatty acids, meaning: no double bond or one or more double bonds.

Since saturated fatty acids have a linear molecular structure, they are more stable and are needed for structures that require more support. The unsaturated fatty acids have one or more double bonds and are not as stable but, in turn, are more flexible and elastic. They adjust perfectly to fluctuating structures (e.g. cell membranes, genetic link-

ages). However, because they are so flexible, they are also more susceptible to damage from oxidation (see oxidative stress) and other harmful substances. This is why it is so important to protect them against such damage with micronutrients and antioxidants.

There are short-chain fatty acids with 4 carbon atoms per chain, medium-chain fatty acids with up to 12 carbon atoms, and long-chain fatty acids with more than 12 carbon atoms per chain.

Omega-3 fatty acids are called such because their double bond is at the third carbon atom from the end of the carbon chain (Omega is the final letter of the Greek alphabet).

Omega-6 fatty acids have a double bond at the 6th carbon atom from the end.

Cis- or Trans-fatty acids get their respective names depending on whether the remainder of the molecules are situated on the same side (Cis) or on the opposite side (Trans) of the double bond.

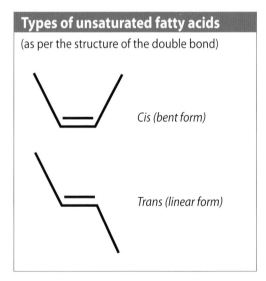

Types of unsaturated fatty acids
(as per the structure of the double bond)

Cis (bent form)

Trans (linear form)

As mentioned before, Trans-fatty acids are somewhat harmful to our body because they promote insulin resistance (which causes weight gain) and LDL-cholesterol (arteriosclerosis factor). Cis-fatty acids are better and healthier for our body (only if we do not convert them into Trans-fatty acids by frying on too high a heat). They are plentiful in plant oils.

Now let us go back to the Omega-3 fatty acids. As we have learned from the Inuit study, the two most important ones are:

Docosahexaenoic acid (DHA) and Eicosapentaenoic acid (EPA). This is Greek and means:

➡ Docos 22 and Hexa 6

➡ Eicos 20 and Penta 5

DHA means a fatty acid with 22 carbon atoms and 6 double bonds and EPA means a fatty acid with 20 carbon atoms and 5 double bonds, each of them having a double bond at the third carbon atom from the end (Omega-3 fatty acid).

DHA is synthesized through EPA which, in turn, has to come from food. An adult produces less than 1 % of alpha-linoleic acid by himself.

Now it becomes clear: the short-chain Omega-3 fatty acids of olive oil and linseed oil in the Mediterranean countries have little to do with the long-chain Omega-3 fatty acids consumed by the Inuit. Our body can only produce extremely small quantities of these long-chain fatty acids. This is why it has to be provided through food. We obtain them by eating fatty coldwater fish (salmon, mackerel, sardines, anchovies, krill and some algae) or by taking fish oil capsules as nutritional supplements.

Wild coldwater fish as a source of Omega-3 fatty acids are better than fish oil capsules because the warm water at fish farms causes the DHA and EPA to decrease in the fish. The need for flexible muscle and vascular structures in cold water is not as high for warm water fish. This is why fish from warm water have fewer fatty acids.

Unfortunately, the increasing pollution of our oceans will make it impossible in the future to easily obtain such fish-derived fatty acids for our body. And giving corn as feed to farmed salmon is not favorable for the content of DHA/EPA in the fish either. (Did you ever see a salmon in a field nibbling on a corncob?) Even the oil in fish oil capsules has to come from wild coldwater fish because the risk of contamination from antibiotics, growth hormones and antifungal substances from farmed fish is too great.

However the effect on our body is even greater.

DHA/EPA has an anti-inflammatory and vasodilating effect on our body. Omega-6 fatty acids are responsible for inflammation and vasoconstriction. Both are necessary, however in reasonable proportion to each other. If, however, both fatty acids use the same enzyme for their metabolism but the DHA/EPA part is constantly decreasing

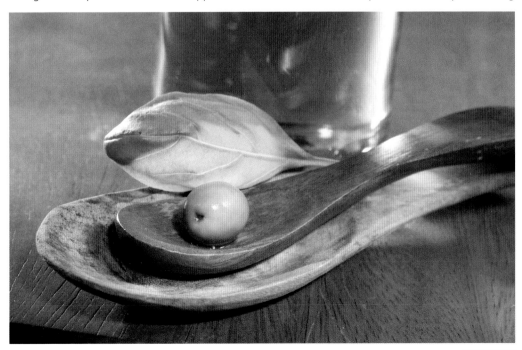

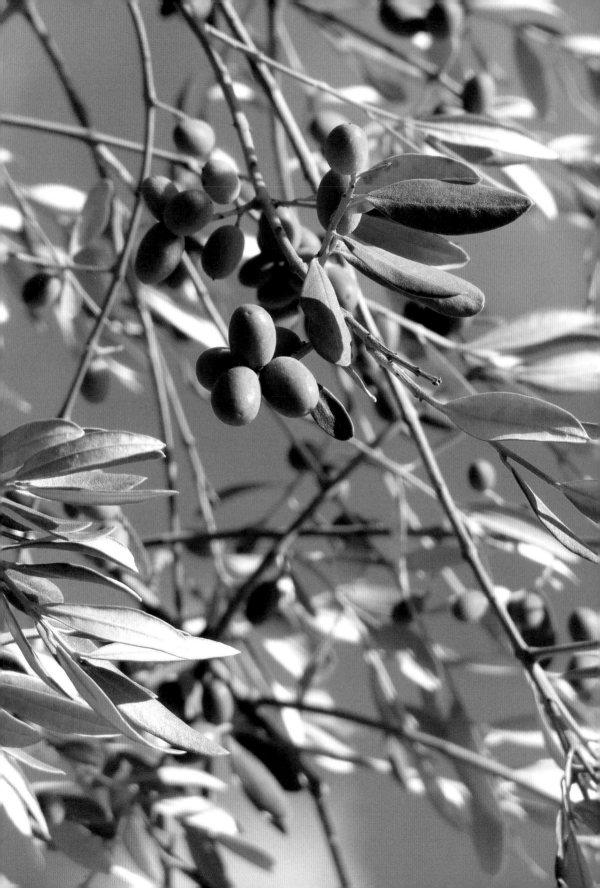

(because the intake from food has been insufficient and the body is unable to produce enough on its own) then an imbalance in both fatty acid groups and its consequences is inevitable. Currently a ratio of 4:1 of Omega-6 to Omega-3 fatty acids is recommended. The ratio, however, in our diet is 32:1.

It has been proven that a balanced ratio of Omega-6 to Omega-3 fatty acids has a positive effect on lowering blood pressure, preventing arteriosclerosis and thus heart attack and stroke. The flow properties of blood are also influenced in a positive way because the red blood cells and the walls of the vessels become more flexible which, in turn, improves the blood and oxygen supply to the brain, heart and other tissues.

DHA plays a major role in the development of the brain and the retina, a reason why it is increasingly administered to pregnant women and toddlers. The mammary glands of the mother are human tissue that is capable of synthesizing DHA to breast milk and thus is very favorable for a baby's brain development. Cow's milk does not contain DHA!

The anti-inflammatory effect on chronic inflammatory and autoimmune diseases is well documented. The increasingly produced Ecosanoids of the Omega-3 fatty acids are our allies which put a stop to the bad Eicosanoids of the Omega-6 fatty acids.

DHA and EPA play a major role in new research on depression. Their influence on the neurotransmitters Serotonin and Dopamine seems to be the main factor and its success is statistically well corroborated.

Other scientific studies regarding schizophrenia, AD(H)S, dementia and other neurodegenerative disorders confirm that the role of DHA and EPA is becoming increasingly more important.

Note: It should be understood that a supply of nutritional supplements alone cannot act as a panacea. A supportive healthy mental and emotional environment during our development cannot be substituted by a few nutritional molecules.

Of course the supply of Omega-3 fatty acids will depend on the needs of the body. A daily amount between 0.04 and 0.1 oz is recommended, depending on body weight. It is advisable to take a sufficient amount of Omega-3 fatty acids for life.

The basics for the 21 Day Metabolic Diet:
➡ A regular supply from coldwater fish from controlled catches
➡ A supply of anti-oxidative nutrients from vegetables, salads and raw food to avoid the unnecessary enzymatic drain on Omega-3 fatty acids
➡ Fish oil capsules from a high quality source

The easiest way to do pillar 6:
➡ In the morning and in the evening take fish oil capsules with nutritional supplements from a high quality source.

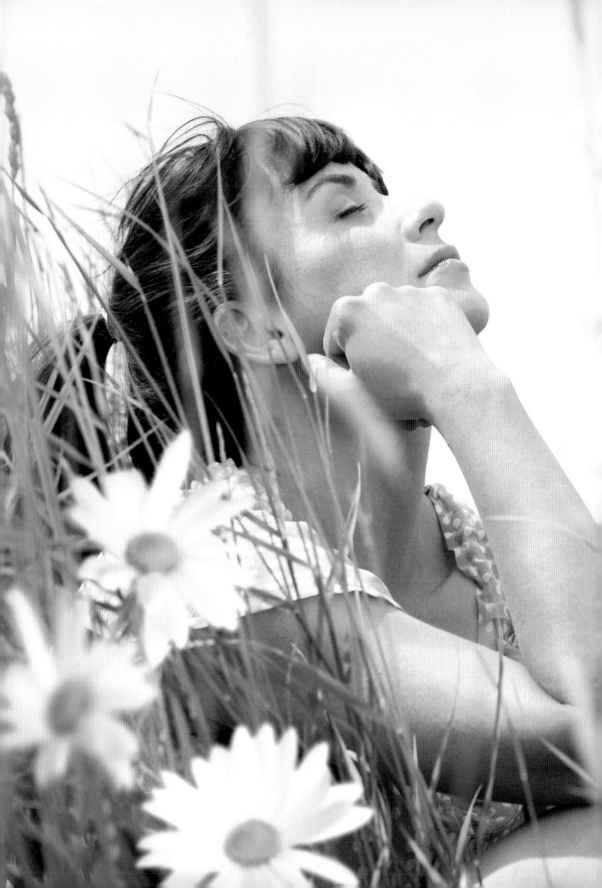

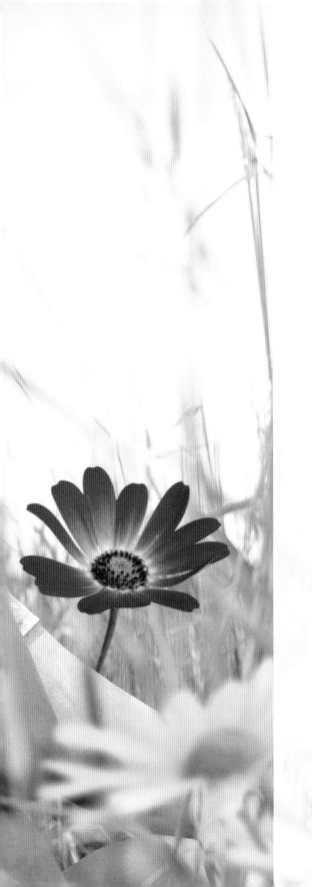

PILLAR 7
Rebalance your metabolism
IN 21 DAYS

**INNER COMPOSURE SUCCESS
THROUGH FEELING,
MIND AND BODY**

7) INNER COMPOSURE SUCCESS THROUGH FEELING, MIND AND BODY

Please think about the following three terms: child, ball, car.

You may still remember this from school as the subject of an essay and, in no time, you have the makings of a story. A child plays with a ball, does not pay attention, a car comes along...

We cannot help ourselves. We automatically tell ourselves a story and find an explanation that makes the past compatible with the experiences of our life to date. Personal experiences or simply general, socially acknowledged convictions that we have adopted throughout the course of our lives, picked up from our parents, teachers, friends or other people that are important to us.

We react to each (new or repetitive) situation with an almost knee-jerk response and create an explanation pattern that then expresses itself as a sensation, inner composure and matching conviction – something that will often show on the outside as a certain attitude. And this feeling, inner and outer attitude, in turn, makes it easier for us to find information, proof and examples that corroborate our story. We find examples and explanations which make our story plausible and understandable. Our brain has no choice but to react in this way. It is made like that because it helps to make situations easy to explain. This helps us save precious time that would be lost if we had to think too long about things. In this way, we can make almost instantaneous decisions and are able to react when necessary. And this is a good thing.

If you are facing a saber-toothed tiger and think you need to pet it first, measure the length of its teeth and check its claws before you are sure that it really is a dangerous animal, then it will probably be too late. We are certainly not descendants of this kind of human. This is why falling back on conclusive explanations that help with decision making in dangerous situations has been a proven system over the course of evolution.

Unfortunately, our brain reacts in the same way even when there is no danger and we could actually embark on a new experience that would allow us to move forward. From an evolutionary standpoint, it made better survival sense to escape from imminent danger instead of experiencing something new to expand one´s horizons. When it comes to weighing up new situations, we tend to revert to the preferred tried and tested methods. This, however, can also restrict our development.

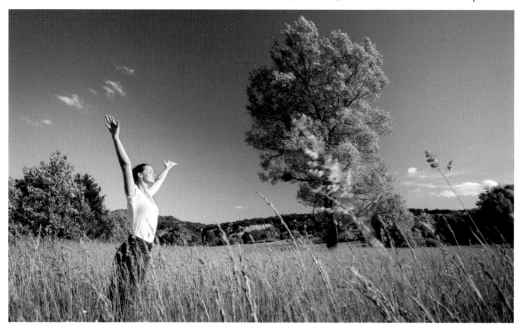

As children we are still open to new experiences and engage in each new event with wonder. We learn by imitation and do not allow failure to stop us from continuing to practice. When a child begins to walk, it walks because of its need to imitate the people around it because everyone else walks on two legs and is not crawling on all fours. Even after the fifth or tenth or hundredth attempt, the child still does not give up but keeps on practicing until it can stand. We have all done this otherwise we would still be crawling. Only during the course of our lives do we lose this steadfast confidence in our skills and often justify stopping with the following sentences – our so called "set of beliefs":

MEMO:

Dare to fail and make mistakes, they are part of life.

Later you will regret the things you have never done.

➡ It´s not going to work anyway!

➡ I´ve tried everything already!

➡ My body always reacts differently!

➡ It doesn´t help anyway!

➡ It won't last anyway!

If we approach something new with this old set of beliefs, we sabotage our success from the very beginning. Each and every one of our actions is overshadowed by a fear of failure and will be carried out halfheartedly and if it really turns out to be a failure, this just confirms our initial conviction. And now something awful happens: our reward system in the brain becomes very active and releases endorphins, the so-called "happiness hormones" – we were right from the get go!

This is how we can keep on living comfortably from one failure to the next…

And yes! Of course, you have already found that diets do not work. And yes, you tried many diets and your body did react in a different way from everyone else. And yes, of course you have heard from many people in your social circle that this does not really help and works only for a short while!

And yes, this does happen! Our everyday life and our behavior have become so complicated with all the decisions, insecurities and uncertainties with which we are faced that all these results are possible and unpredictable. This is the fullness and unplanned arbitrariness of our life.

And yes! For the result you want to achieve, because it is important to you, you just have to get up one more time and try it once more, despite your previous experiences…

…and now open yourself up to new things and allow the chance of succeeding to enter into your thinking and feeling. There is just the possibility that it might work after everything you have tried, that you will be successful just like you always hoped. Imagine at any time of the day that you are already how you would like to be: in the morning, at midday and in the evening. How you will walk, sit, laugh, dress, everything – as if it were already a reality…

Be a child again and have the confidence to be able "to stand up and walk" because this skill lies naturally within us. The journey up to the point where we can "stand up and walk" with all its experiences is very personal. For some it will be shorter for others longer. However not a single step, no experience will have been in vain. All of them were important to you on your journey to success.

Have new experiences. Take a few risks like a child that finally wants to stand up and walk – with a smile, a little anger, with doubts, with wonder, with excitement and a little fear of stumbling. All this is part of such a journey. It is a part of you – and this is a good thing!

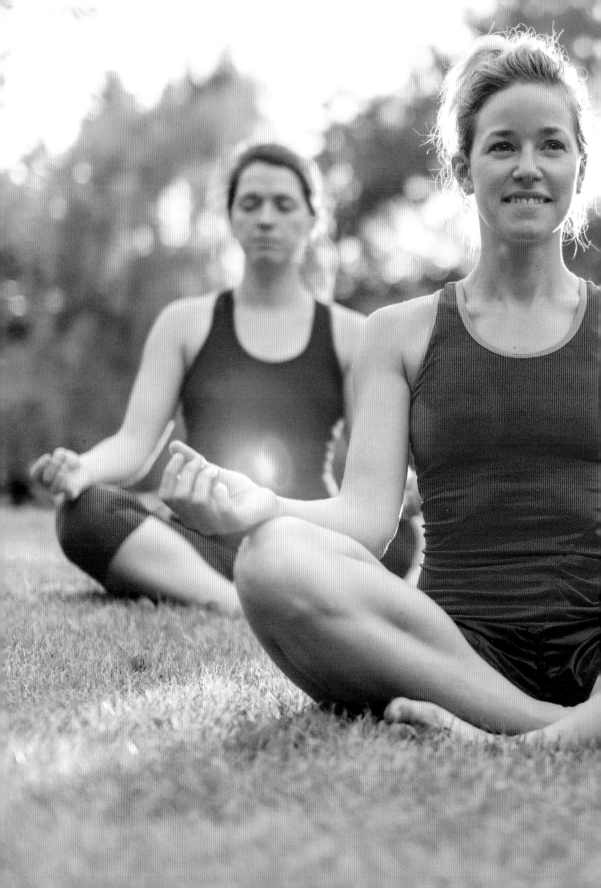

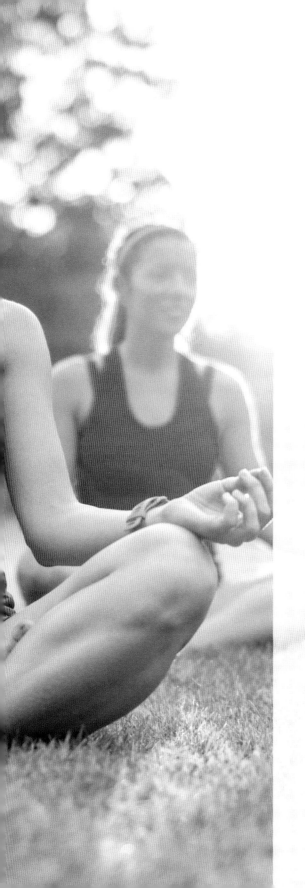

Rebalance your metabolism
IN 21 DAYS

THE CATALYST FOR FAT LOSS AND METABOLIC TRAINING

The Catalyst for Fat Loss and Metabolic Training

The only place where fat deposits can be burned is in our muscles. The more we use our muscles, the more fat can be metabolized. Four factors determine the percentage of muscle mass to body weight: 1. Genetics, 2. Gender, 3. Age and 4. Physical activity.

True, we cannot influence those first three factors. In fact, by virtue of genetics, men have more muscle mass than women. This is why, in most cases, men burn more calories than women despite the same body weight. From the age of 30 onwards, the body loses about 6.5 lbs of active muscle mass every 10 years. As a result, not only do we lose strength and speed, but our metabolic rate decreases as well.

Fortunately, not only are we able to stop this process, but actually reverse it, thanks to factor no. 4.

Numerous studies have proven that the percentage of muscle mass can be increased well into old age by taking the appropriate measures. This enables us at any age to increase our metabolism and energy consumption. In this regard, we have to distinguish between the energy required at rest, which is our base metabolic rate, and the energy required when physically or mentally active, our so-called active metabolic rate.

The base metabolic rate runs 24 hours a day and normally uses over 70 % of the body's entire energy consumption. By increasing the percentage of active muscles, both the base metabolic rate and the active metabolic rate increase and thus more fat is burned.

The more muscle, the higher the base metabolic rate. The higher the base metabolic rate, the more energy used

This diagram shows two women.
The woman on the right has 22.5 lbs more muscle mass.
The woman on the left has 22.5 lbs more body fat.

Body weight	132.0 lbs	132.0 lbs
Percentage of body fat	35 %	18 %
Body fat	46.2 lbs	23.8 lbs
Lean body mass*	85.8 lbs	108.2 lbs
Base metabolic rate	**1,211 kcal**	**1,433 kcal**

* (Only muscles burn fat)

What is required, as far as body weight is concerned, to increase the percentage of active muscles and thus burn more fat?

The only way of obtaining this is by specific resistance training. That requires overcoming a resistance in accordance with general training principles. This means that the resistance on the muscles must be controlled in terms of strength, intensity, duration, extent, number of repetitions and the relationship between stress and recovery.

For best results, it is useful to seek professional help e.g. at a good fitness or health center. Circuit training, which can provide stress parameters and rest times, is highly efficient with a minimal investment in time. Two 30 minute training sessions per week are enough to increase the metabolism and keep it at a consistently higher level. This is a perfect metabolic workout. It has been proven that endurance training will not have the same effect.

The metabolic training program during the metabolic diet

Since we deprive our body of carbohydrates and fats while on the metabolic diet, our body takes advantage of any free fatty acids. In order to function normally, our body has to compensate for the increased energy consumption caused by the metabolic training program by releasing a large amount of fatty acids from stored fat. This way, we can significantly enhance the effect of the metabolic diet as far as the breakdown of unwanted fat deposits is concerned.

Furthermore, it has been proven that an increase in muscle mass leads, amongst other things, to positive effects on the cardio-vascular system, the psyche, the skin, the immune system, bone density and blood sugar levels.

NOTE:

Good performance depends on our circulation. Have a mixed drink containing amino acids and vitamins to encourage better physical performance. Vitamin C supports the blood vessels and counteracts exhaustion and fatigue. The drink should also contain a concentrate of L-Arginin.

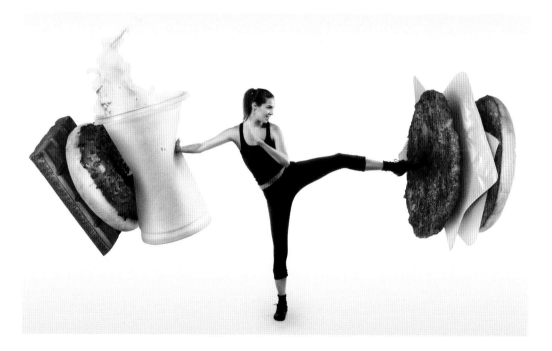

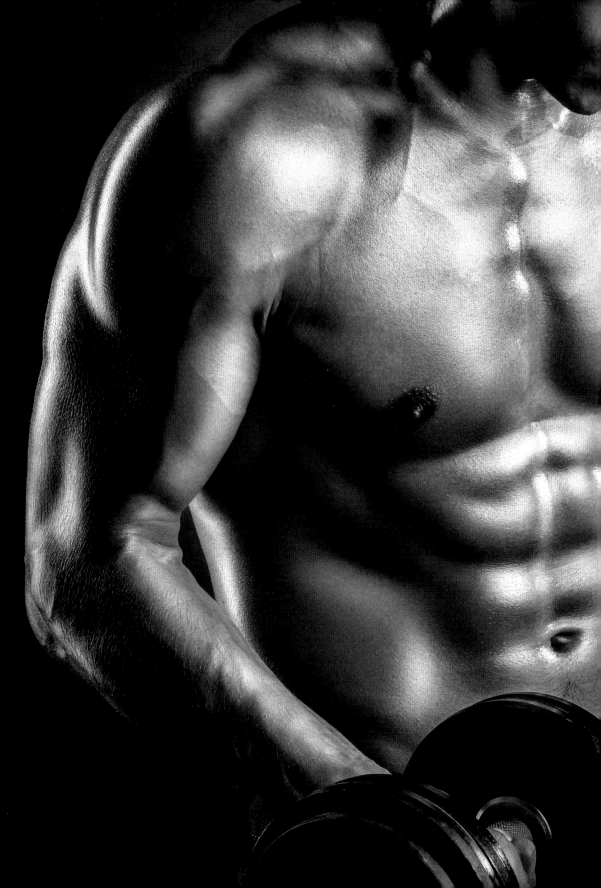

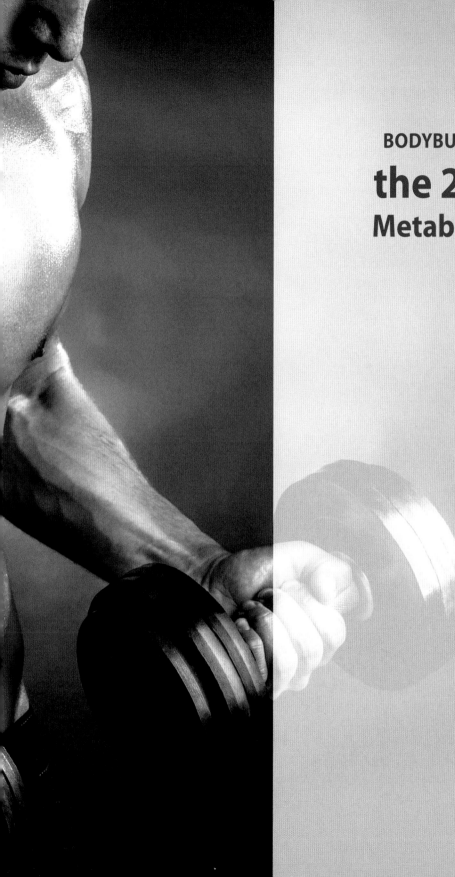

BODYBUILDING AND

the 21 Day
Metabolic Diet

Bodybuilding and the 21 Day Metabolic Diet

For a long time I have been thinking about whether we should include the subject "Metabolic Diet for bodybuilders". However, since I have been asked many times how a bodybuilder who wants to reduce body fat but not muscles, could use the metabolic diet, I have included some experiences from my practice.

First of all, I would like to note that everything I am writing here is based on experiences I have had with people during the course of mentoring them while on the diet. Up until now, there have been no clinical studies as to what professional body-builders/strength training athletes should eat. I have practiced intensive bodybuilding myself for almost 15 years and participated in many competitions. The metabolic diet is perfect for losing stored body fat without losing muscle – it is ideal for bodybuilders.

Every strength training athlete/bodybuilder should adjust their caloric intake during the course of their training regime (where possible in consultation with their doctor or trainer) in such a way that they can reach their desired result. When an athlete wants to reduce body fat, it is not possible to build up muscle naturally at the same time – in ideal circumstances, muscle mass, at the most, can only be maintained.

At the same time, training in the maximum power zone, especially in the field of endurance, is difficult. Please keep in mind that insulin is always needed to open the cells of the muscles. As our carbohydrate intake is minimal during the metabolic diet, insulin production is very low at this time.

In a nutshell, as I stated above, the 21-day metabolic diet is highly suitable for bodybuilders/strength training athletes for reducing stored body fat. As described in previous chapters, the decrease in energy caused by the low caloric intake has only a minimal or no influence on performance because of the supporting effect of homeopathy and the right kind of micronutrients.

We know that fat burn-off only takes place if the energy supply is less than the energy consumed. The actual difference in a professional bodybuilder as compared to the general population is that their base metabolic rate is so much higher due to their greater muscle mass. I have measured the base metabolic rate of professional bodybuilders up to 4,500 kcal.

The base metabolic rate of a normal bodybuilder is expected to be approximately 2,500 to 3,000 kcal. If we include their active metabolic rate and their training, we quickly reach a daily need for 3,500 kcal or more. Since the normal diet plan of the 21-day metabolic diet provides approximately 600 – 700 kcal, I recommend adjusting the caloric intake on an individual basis. A bodybuilder who needs, for example, 3,500 kcal can double or even triple his caloric intake. He will then be provided with a total caloric supply of approximately 2,000 kcal.

From our own experience, we know that the diet works perfectly with a caloric deficiency of 2,000 kcal. It is important that you keep to the selection of foods listed on the plan. My own blood results and those of my clients were not significantly changed by the increase in protein.

NOTE:

Again the same applies: please speak with your trainer or doctor. Experience with our clients has shown that there was only a minimal amount of muscle loss, as long as they adhered closely to the diet plan.

My co-author Christian Mörwald is 48 years old, 5 ft 6 in and a keen sportsman with regular 45 minute weight training 3 times a week and 45 minute cardio training 1-2 times a week. This means he is not considered a professional athlete. He experimented by doubling his energy supply to an average of approximately 1,330 kcal/day and with more protein to find out how this would affect his diet results. His body weight reduced from 162.8lbs to 152.9 lbs and the percentage of body fat decreased from 18 % to 12.5 %.

Example of a nutrition protocol for one day:

Time	Amount (oz)	Food	Energy (kcal)	Protein (oz)
6:00 am	2	95 % protein concentrate	195.5	1.67
1:00 pm		Minced beef (see recipe part):		
	10-1/2	Lean beef minced	339.0	2.22
	2	Onion	14.0	0.02
	1 tbsp	Dijon Mustard	15.3	0.03
	1-1/2 tbsp	Tomato purée	11.1	0.02
	2 tbsp	Dried tomatoes	30.0	0.06
	1 tbsp	Dried peppers	21.3	0.05
	7	Sieved tomatoes	34.0	0.07
	0.035	Pepper	3.0	0.003
	1 tbsp	Parsley	5.3	0.014
		Salt		
		Vegetables:		
	10-1/2	Brussels sprouts	84.0	0.42
	1 tbsp	Vegetable stock	11.2	0.0
5:30 pm	2	95 % Protein concentrate	195.5	1.67
10:30 pm		Mixed salad with tuna:		
	10	Tuna in water, drained	274.4	2.27
	10-1/2	Iceberg salad	39.0	0.11
	14	Cucumber	48.0	0.14
	7	Tomato	34.0	0.07
	7	Sweet peppers, yellow	60.0	0.07
	2	Balsamic vinegar	44.0	0.02
	2 tbsp	Chives	5.4	0.03
Liquids Per day	92 oz/2-3/4 qts	Water	0.4	0.0
	16 oz/1/2 qt	Coffee black	10.0	0.0
		Total	**1.474,0**	**8,96**

Note: Contrary to the recommendation of the DGE (German Association for Nutrition) to limit the daily intake of protein to 0.07 oz per 2.2 lbs body weight, Christian Mörwald has been taking 7 oz – 10.5 oz of protein for about 25 years.

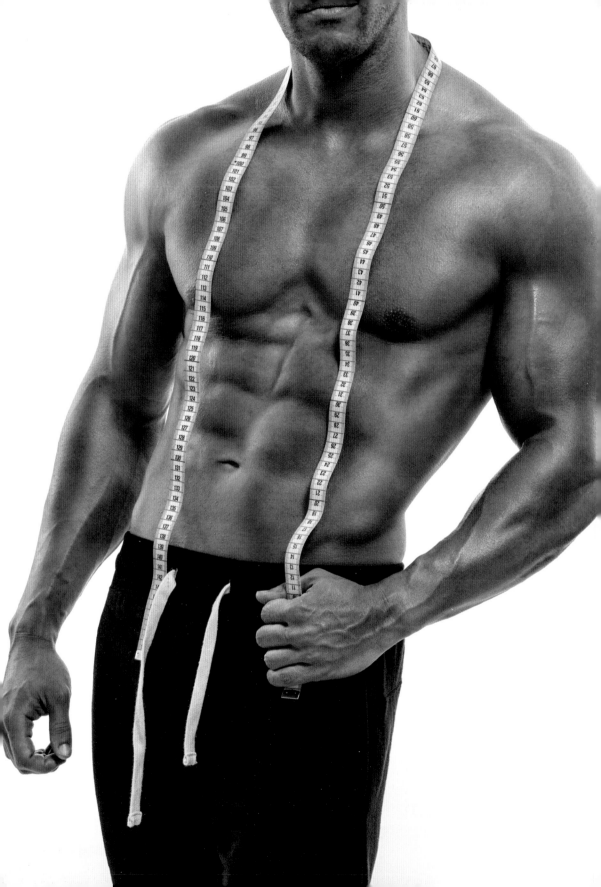

Course of the Diet

	Weight (lbs)	Fat (%)	Fat (lbs)	Visceral fat	Lean Build (lbs)	Energy (kcal)	Protein (oz)
Loading Day 1	**163**	**18.0**	**29**	**9**	**134**		
Loading Day 2							
Diet Day 1	166	15.6	26	9	140	1,073	7.05
Diet Day 2	163	16.8	27	9	136	1,006	6.77
Diet Day 3	161	18.4	30	9	131	1.065	6.84
Diet Day 4	162	17.7	29	9	133	1,047	6.81
Diet Day 5	160	19.0	30	8	129	1.234	8.43
Diet Day 6	159	16.7	27	8	133	1,313	8.25
Diet Day 7	160	16.1	26	8	134	1,249	8.61
Diet Day 8	159	15.5	25	8	134	1,302	7.48
Diet Day 9						1,466	8.92
Diet Day 10	157	16.5	26	8	131	1,247	6.70
Diet Day 11	157	15.3	24	8	133	1,252	7.80
Diet Day 12	157	15.8	25	8	132	1,405	7.76
Diet Day13	70.7	15.0	23	7	132	1,281	8.22
Diet Day 14						1,450	7.51
Diet Day 15	156	12.9	20	7	136	1,410	7.55
Diet Day 16	156	14.5	23	8	133	1,489	8.36
Diet Day 17	155	14.8	23	7	132	1,400	7.62
Diet Day 18	154	14.5	22	7	132	1,452	8.85
Diet Day 19						1,520	9.03
Diet Day 20	154	14.1	22	7	132	1,601	8.04
Diet Day 21	152	14.6	22	7	130	1,350	7.48
Stabilization Day 1					1,518	8.75	
Stabilization Day 2	153	14.9	23	7	130	1,499	8.18
Stabilization Day 3	153	12.5	21	7	132		
Total						30.604	
Average						**1,331**	**7.90**

One of my highly performance-oriented clients (45-60 minute stationary bicycle workout in the morning 4 – 5 times a week plus strength training in the evening 4 times a week) who modified the diet by tripling his energy supply and increasing his protein intake, reported that during the 21 diet days he lost 17lbs 10 oz of fat while his performance was unaffected during the training.

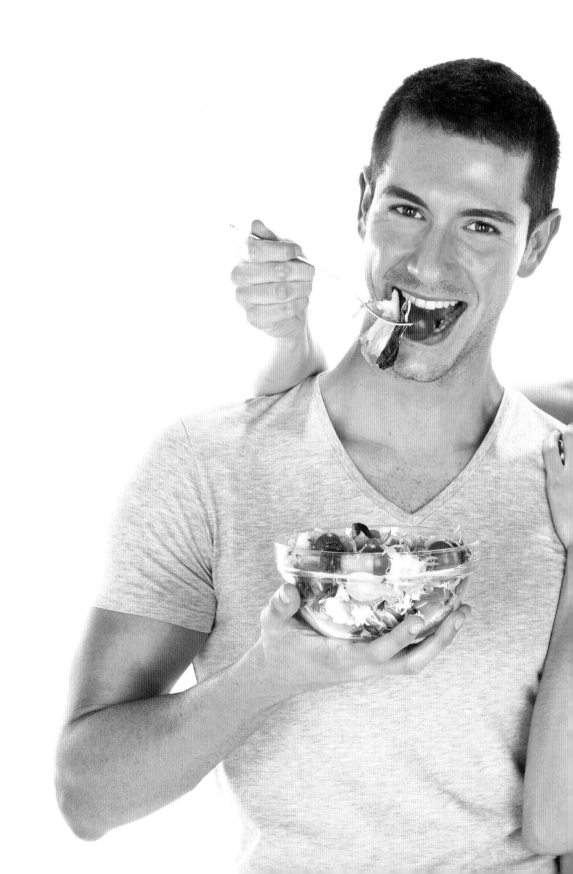

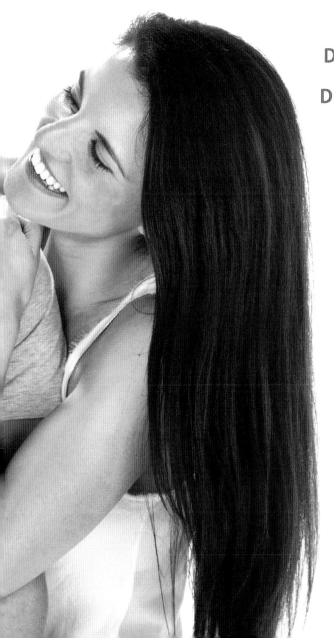

RECIPES TO
rebalance your metabolism
IN 21 DAYS

DELICIOUS DISHES FOR THE

DIET PHASE, STABILIZATION
PHASE AND TEST PHASE

STABILIZATION PHASE
AND TEST PHASE

TEST PHASE

Nutritional facts

The nutritional values listed have been carefully researched. They are based on the average values indicated by the manufacturer and various nutritional charts and reference books.

With these indicators you will be able to tailor the ingredients of our delicious recipes to fit your individual needs.

Explanation of the abbreviations:

Kcal = kilocalories (1kcal = 4.184 Kilojoules)
P   = Protein
C   = Carbohydrate
F   = Fat

If we give you a choice of ingredients (e.g. 7oz ricotta or low fat quark) our nutritional values refer to the first ingredient.

Individual energy requirements

The following information is just meant as a rough guide. There is no formula with which you can calculate the exact caloric requirements for each person.

The caloric requirements comprise the base metabolic rate and the active metabolic rate.

The **base metabolic rate** is the amount of calories your body needs at rest.

A simple formula to estimate the base metabolic rate:

Men: 10.9 kcal x body weight in lbs per day
Women: 9.8 kcal x body weight in lbs per day

A more precise calculation taking into consideration body composition:

(370 + (9.8 x lean body mass in lbs) kcal per day

> **NOTE:**
>
> The higher the percentage of lean muscle mass (i.e. the lower the percentage of fat), the higher the base metabolic rate and the more you need to eat.
>
> Muscle weighs more than fat. This means that the higher the percentage of muscle and the lower the percentage of fat, the leaner the body, despite weighing the same.

The **active metabolic rate** is the energy your body needs to carry out your daily activities. It basically depends on your base metabolic rate and the kind of activities you perform.

For a simple and quick assessment of the active metabolic rate, you can apply the so-called PAL factor (Physical Activity Level). It divides people into 5 different groups according to their physical activity.

PAL Factor	Activities
1.2	People who have a predominantly sedentary lifestyle (e.g. frail or disabled people)
1.3 – 1.5	People with an almost predominantly sedentary lifestyle and very few leisure activities (e.g. people who work long hours at their desks)
1.6 – 1.7	People who predominantly work in a sedentary position but include a little additional walking / standing activities (e.g. school children, students, truck drivers, lab workers)
1.8 – 1.9	People with predominantly walking / standing activities (e.g. home makers, waiters, workmen, shop assistants
2.0 – 2.4	People with physically demanding activities (e.g. farmers, miners, competitive sports people)

If your daily activities consist of, for example, office work and a quiet evening at home, you can take a PAL factor of 1.4.

Using the PAL factor you can calculate your daily caloric requirements.

Calculation of the caloric requirements for the woman on the left of the diagram on page 66 (85.8 lbs lean body mass)

Base metabolic rate:

(370 + (9.8 x lean body mass in lbs) kcal per day = (370 + (9.8 x 85.8) kcal per day = 1,211 kcal per day

Total caloric requirement:

Base metabolic rate x PAL factor = 1,211 x 1.4 = 1,695 kcal

The following chart may be useful as a reference for the caloric requirements for different activities. It shows the approximate calorie consumption of 154 – 176 lbs.

Activity	Calorie consumption
Sleeping	60
Sitting	80
Standing	120
Going for a walk	280
Playing golf	360
Playing tennis	450
Fitness training	480
Walking	520
Climbing steps	560
Playing soccer	700
Cycling at 15.5 miles/hr	820
Bodybuilding	820
Mountain hiking with backpack	880
Jogging at 7.5 miles/hr	1000

RECIPES FOR THE DIET PHASE, STABILIZATION PHASE AND TEST PHASE

Breakfast variations

The morning shake consists of two components:

➡ Protein shake, aspartame free (one portion approx. 1 oz, nutritional value: approx. 88 kcal, 350 KJ), 0 oz F, 0.039 oz C, 0.78 oz P)

➡ Comprehensive nutritional supplement with fiber (2 scoops)

The protein shake is important to support muscle and lean body mass (so as to avoid muscle loss). Furthermore, it is satisfying and does not leave you hungry. During the diet phase mix the shake with water. Afterwards feel free to mix it with skim milk.

This comprehensive nutritional supplement is the basis for a successful diet. In a way it is your fruit and vegetables out of a container with no chemicals or additives. It provides vitamins, minerals and trace elements which help to maintain a correct pH balance. The added fiber swells in your stomach and also provides you with a feeling of satisfaction. Fiber helps to cleanse the intestines.

There are two ways of preparing these two items:

➡ Mix them together or

➡ Take them separately

Variations

➡ Breakfast "porridge" to eat with a spoon

Put a little less water in the shaker and shake until the liquid thickens to a Cream of Wheat or porridge-like consistency. Add cinnamon and stevia if you like. Tip into a breakfast bowl and eat with a spoon…Delicious! Don´t forget to drink a lot of water.

➡ Shake with cold tea

Use one of the teas from the list of "allowed beverages" and allow it to cool (add stevia to taste if you like). Drink immediately as it quickly becomes thick.

➡ Mix shake with vitamin drink e.g. from Lifeplus

The orange flavored vitamin drink is very good for encouraging weight loss during the diet. (It is an excellent support during the diet phase).

➡ For coffee drinkers

Pour one cup of cold coffee into the shaker and add 1-1/3 cups of water.

Add triple protein shake and mix with 2 scoops of vitamin powder. Delicious!

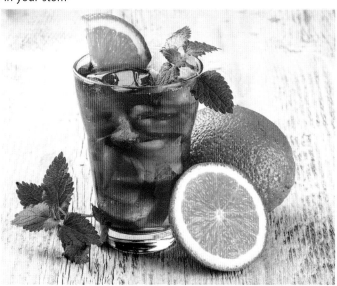

The following ingredients are just guidelines. E.g. during the diet phase vegetables and salads are unlimited but proteins are limited to 4 oz or 4-1/2 oz per meal.

DIET PHASE – STABILIZATION PHASE – TEST PHASE

Fish Filet with Mediterranean Vegetables

Ingredients:

5 oz	Fish filet of choice
4 oz	Onions
6 tbsp	Vegetable stock without MSG
2	Bell peppers red/yellow
8 oz	Tomatoes
5 oz	Zucchini
2 tbsp	Fresh herbs (e.g. thyme, parsley)
	Rock salt and black pepper
1	Lemon

Nutritional values

Approx. total
325 kcal
(1360 kJ)
0.14 oz F
1.13 oz C
1.27 oz P

Preparation:

Season the fish filet with salt and lemon and set aside. Peel the onions, cut in half and slice thinly then sauté in a little water. Wash and dice the bell peppers, add to onions and sauté for 5 minutes. Cut the zucchini in half and slice. Add the tomatoes and stock. Season with salt and pepper. Fry the fish in a non-stick pan. Finely chop the herbs and add to the vegetables. Simmer for 7 minutes on a medium heat. Arrange the vegetables and fish on a plate and drizzle with lemon juice.

Chicken Curry with Green Asparagus

Ingredients:

5 oz	Chicken breast filets
10 spears	Green asparagus
1 head	Lettuce
1	Large tomato
1	Onion
1	Lemon
	Curry powder, sea salt, black pepper
1/2 oz	Fresh ginger

Nutritional values

Approx. total
271 kcal
(1134 kJ)
0.07 oz F
0.56 oz C
1.55 oz P

Preparation:

Slice the chicken breast into filets and season with the salt, pepper and curry. Peel the ginger, chop finely and rub on the chicken filets. Marinate for 20 minutes.

Cut the asparagus into 2-inch pieces. Peel the onion and finely dice. Finely dice the tomato.

Arrange the salad leaves on a platter, drizzle with lemon juice and season with salt and pepper. In a non-stick pan, fry the chicken filets.

Add the asparagus and diced onions. Season with salt and pepper.

Just before removing the chicken from the pan, add the tomato pieces and quickly stir fry for one minute. Place everything on top of the salad, drizzle with lemon juice, season with salt and pepper.

DIET PHASE – STABILIZATION PHASE – TEST PHASE

Cauliflower Meatloaf

Nutritional values	
Approx. total	1384 kcal
	(5786 kJ)
	1.48 oz F
	0.71 oz C
	7.87 oz P

Ingredients:

1	Cauliflower
Approx. 2 lbs	lean hamburger (depending on the size of the cauliflower)
	Salt, pepper, mustard without sugar
1-2	Onions
1 tsp	Vegetable stock without MSG
	Herbs to taste, e.g. parsley

Preparation:

Cook cauliflower in the vegetable stock for approximately 10 minutes and allow to cool. Season the hamburger meat with salt, pepper, mustard, onions and parsley.

Next spread the hamburger mixture over the cauliflower. The cauliflower should be completely covered.

Bake for 50 min. at 300º F. Then increase the heat to 400º F and allow to brown for approximately 10 minutes.

TIP:

In the stabilization phase the cauliflower covered in hamburger can also be wrapped with 7 oz of bacon or slices of smoked turkey breast. Simply wrap the cauliflower with the hamburger as described above and spread the bacon or smoked turkey breast over it making sure there is only one layer of bacon or smoked turkey breast. The cauliflower and the hamburger should be completely covered.

Bake for 50 min. at 300º F and then allow to brown for about another 10 minutes.

Spicy Mushrooms au gratin

Nutritional values	
Approx. total	165 kcal
	(690 kJ)
	0.04 oz F
	0.14 oz C
	1.23 oz P

Ingredients

12	Mushrooms
4 oz	Harzer cheese or another low fat cheese
1	Onion
	Pepper

Preparation:

Pre-heat oven to 350º F.

Clean the mushrooms, remove the stems, and set aside. Peel and chop the onion. Chop the mushroom stems. Place the mushrooms in a small casserole dish. Spread chopped onions over the mushrooms. Cut the Harzer/low fat cheese into 12 pieces and place on top of the mushrooms. Season with pepper and bake for approximately 10 minutes.

DIET PHASE – STABILIZATION PHASE – TEST PHASE

Hamburgers

Ingredients:

2 lbs	Lean hamburger
1-2	Onions
3-4 tsp	Mustard without sugar
3-4 tsp	Tomato paste
2 oz	Sun dried tomatoes
1 oz	Dried peppers
	Freshly ground pepper
1-1/4lbs	Sieved tomatoes (Passata)

Nutritional values

Approx. total
1582 kcal
(6619 kJ)
1.80 oz F
1.52 oz C
8.04 oz P

Preparation:

Put onions, sun dried tomatoes and peppers in an electric food processor.

Add this mixture to the hamburger. Now add the mustard, tomato paste and pepper. Make hamburgers from this mixture and place in a non-stick casserole dish. Put in the oven for 20-20 minutes at 400° F until brown.

Take the hamburgers out of the casserole dish. Add the sieved tomatoes with the juice for the sauce.

Vegetable Stir Fry

Ingredients:

3	Zucchini
14 oz	Mushrooms
3	Tomatoes
1	Bell pepper
	Pepper, thyme
1 cup	Sieved tomatoes (Passata)

Nutritional values

Approx. total
318 kcal
(1330 kJ)
0.18 oz F
1.27 oz C
1.20 oz P

Preparation:

Wash and chop the vegetables. Stir fry them in a non-stick pan and deglaze with the sieved tomatoes. Season the vegetable stir-fry with pepper and thyme. Delicious, for example, with a piece of turkey from the grill.

DIET PHASE – STABILIZATION PHASE – TEST PHASE

Grilled Pike

Nutritional values

Ingredients:

		Approx. total
9 oz	Fresh pike	227 kcal
1	Lemon	(953 kJ)
1 sprig	Fresh thyme	0.07 oz F
1 pinch	Salt and pepper	0.14 oz C
		1.62 oz P

Preparation:

Wash the pike. Cut half the lemon into slices and juice the other half. Place the pike on a large sheet of aluminum foil.

Stuff the pike with the lemon slices and thyme. Season with salt and pepper. Next wrap the pike and seal the foil. Place the foil package on the barbecue and cook for 5 minutes on each side or cook for 15 minutes in the oven at 400° F.

Cabbage Soup

Nutritional values

Ingredients:

		Approx. total
5 oz	Lean hamburger	380 kcal
14 oz	White cabbage	(1585 kJ)
1 large	Onion	0.28 oz F
1 pc	Fresh ginger	1.16 oz C
1 tsp	Sambal Olek	1.41 oz P
2	Tomatoes	
1 clove	Garlic	
14 oz	Vegetable stock, salt and pepper	

Preparation:

Brown the meat in a pot or pan. Add the finely chopped garlic and ginger.

Cut the cabbage into strips. Dice the tomatoes and onions and add everything to the meat together with the vegetable stock.

Let the soup simmer until the cabbage is soft. Season with salt, pepper and sambal olek.

TIP:

This recipe can be prepared in larger quantities as the soup can be refrigerated for several days. Instead of the hamburger you can also use strips of chicken breast or shrimp.

DIET PHASE – STABILIZATION PHASE – TEST PHASE

Baked Vegetables

Ingredients:

Take vegetables and spices from the list of approved foods
(e.g. mushrooms, zucchini, tomatoes, bell peppers –
choose desired quantity).

Preparation:

Wash and slice the vegetables. Spread the vegetables over a baking tray lined with waxed paper. Season with herbs and spices. Place on the middle rack of the oven and bake for about 35 minutes at 400° F turning the vegetables over once or twice.

TIP:

Delicious with turkey filet from the grill. Choose whatever vegetables and spices you prefer from the approved list.

Steak and Spinach

Nutritional values
Approx. total
237 kcal
(995 kJ)
0.25 oz F
0.21 oz C
1.30 oz P

Ingredients:

5 oz	Steak
5 oz	Fresh or frozen spinach
4 tsp	Non fat vegetable stock (without MSG)
1	Onion
1 clove	Garlic, rock salt, black pepper

Preparation:

Wash the spinach. Peel and dice the onion and garlic. Fry the onions and garlic, add spinach and stir well. Remove from the pan. Fry the steak for about 1 minute on each side (medium). Remove from the pan, season with salt and pepper, cover and leave to rest.

Pour the vegetable stock into the pan, add the spinach and simmer briefly – done!

Arrange everything together on a plate.

DIET PHASE – STABILIZATION PHASE – TEST PHASE

Tomatoes au gratin

Ingredients:

4	Large tomatoes (about 9 oz)
7 oz	Fresh mushrooms
1	Onion
1	Bell pepper
1 lb	Zucchini
7 oz	Harzer cheese or another low fat cheese
	Pepper, ginger, basil, thyme, marjoram

Nutritional values	
Approx. total	
604	kcal
(2527	kJ)
0.25 oz	F
1.83 oz	C
2.93 oz	P

Preparation:

Chop the onion, cut the bell pepper, zucchini into small pieces, slice the mushrooms and stir-fry. Wash the tomatoes, then cut off their tops and scoop out the inside. Place the tomatoes in a casserole dish. Add the rest of the tomato filling to the other vegetables and season with pepper, ginger, basil, thyme and marjoram.

Fill the tomatoes with the vegetable mixture. Dice the cheese finely and spread over the tomatoes. Bake in the oven at 350° F until the cheese has melted.

TIP:

The tomatoes can also be stuffed with shrimp instead of vegetables and then baked with the cheese.

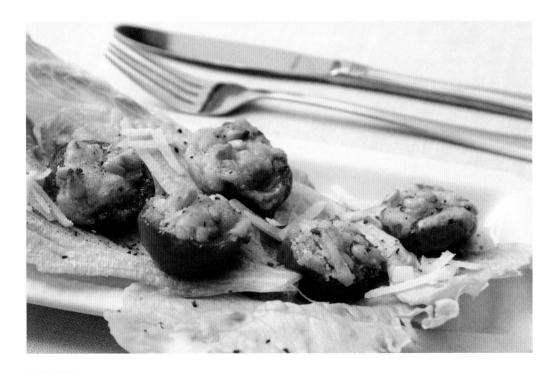

DIET PHASE – STABILIZATION PHASE – TEST PHASE

Vegetarian Vegetable Soup

Ingredients:

1/2	Celery root
2	green and yellow zucchini (one of each)
1-2 tsp	Vegetable stock powder without MSG
5 oz	Swiss chard
1	Bell pepper
	Coriander seeds

Nutritional values

Approx. total
191 kcal
(810 kJ)
0.11 oz F
0.78 oz C
0.56 oz P

Preparation:

Cut the celery root into small pieces to speed up cooking. Cut green and yellow zucchini into slices. Put everything into a pot and cover with enough water to make a soup. Now add the vegetable stock powder and reduce to a simmer as the vegetables will cook very quickly.

Once the celery root is cooked add the Swiss chard and the pepper.

Add spices to taste, if necessary. At the end, add a few coriander seeds for a special flavor. Leave everything on top of the stove until the Swiss chard is cooked.

TIP:

For meat lovers: fry a piece of lean chicken or cod in a non-stick pan and then follow the recipe. Fantastic dish for cooking ahead.

For those who are not on the diet, fry meat/fish in rapeseed, linseed or olive oil. For those who prefer a more exotic flavor, use coconut oil.

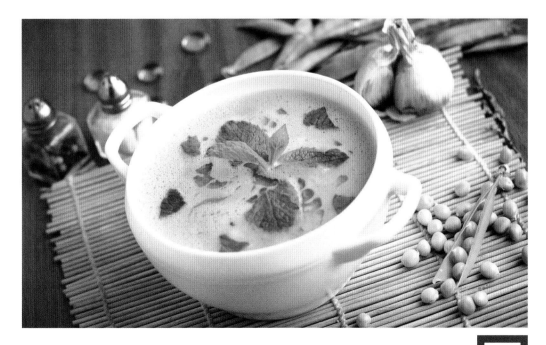

DIET PHASE – STABILIZATION PHASE – TEST PHASE

Zucchini Spaghetti with Lean Hamburger

This recipe serves 4. You can also keep it in the fridge and eat it in 2 days.

Nutritional values

Approx. total
605	kcal
(2545	kJ)
0.53 oz	F
1.38 oz	C
2.68 oz	P

Ingredients:

3-3/4 cups	Vegetable stock
9 oz	Lean hamburger
2	Onions
1 clove	Garlic
1	Red bell pepper (diced)
2	Large tomatoes diced or approximately 8 small tomatoes cut in half
	Tomato paste if desired (sugar-free)
	Spices to taste
4	Zucchini
	Fresh chilli peppers, if desired
1	Spring onion to garnish

Bolognese Sauce:

In a separate pot, bring the vegetable stock to a boil. Fry the hamburger in a non-stick pan until brown. Next add the chopped onions and garlic to the hamburger and sauté until soft. Add the diced pepper and tomatoes and simmer briefly. Reduce the liquid from the vegetables. If you prefer a more liquid sauce, add more stock. Simmer and then add the tomato paste for a creamy texture.

Note: Avoid cooking the peppers and tomatoes for too long so as not to become mushy. Season to taste. Done!

Zucchini Spaghetti:

The zucchini must be prepared just before serving. Put the zucchini in a vegetable spiral cutter to make "spaghetti".

Sauté the zucchini quickly in a frying pan until no longer raw. Remove from heat.

Season with salt arrange on a platter. Ladle on the sauce and garnish with fresh chilli and spring onions.

DIET PHASE – STABILIZATION PHASE – TEST PHASE

Hamburgers with a Bouquet of Salad Greens

Nutritional values

Approx. total
355 kcal
(1500 kJ)
0.28 oz F
0.92 oz C
1.45 oz P

Ingredients:

5 oz	Lean Hamburger
1 small	Red onion
Salad	Mixed seasonal salad leaves: iceberg, lettuce, rocket
1	Red bell pepper
1	Large tomato
1 small	Cucumber
	Mixed herbs
	Balsamic vinegar
	Coarse sea salt, black pepper

Preparation:

Place the hamburger in a bowl. Peel and chop the onions and combine with the hamburger. Add herbs and spices.

Shape into palm size balls and flatten slightly.

Heat the pan and slowly fry the hamburgers on medium heat. To keep the hamburgers juicy, cover the pan with a lid. (Cooking time: 10 minutes.)

At the same time, wash the salad and remove the seeds from the bell pepper.

Tear the salad leaves into small pieces and cut the pepper into thin slices.

Cut the cucumber and tomato into slices. Arrange everything on a platter and dress with herbs, spices and balsamic vinegar.

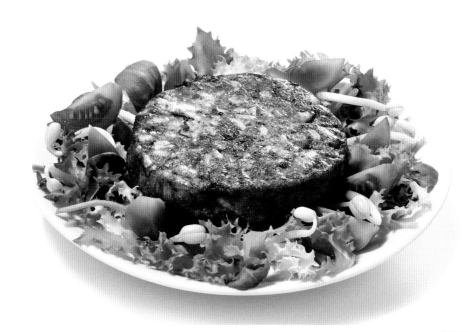

STABILIZATION AND TEST PHASE

Eggplant boats

Turkey medallions with eggplant halves stuffed with spinach, pepper, eggplant and goat's cheese

Nutritional values

Approx. total
1237 kcal
(5521 kJ)
0.32 oz F
0.88 oz C
7.51 oz P

Ingredients:

1	Eggplant
7 oz	Spinach
1	Bell pepper
2	Eggs
6	Turkey medallions
	Coarse black pepper
	Creamy Goat's cheese

Preparation:

Wash eggplant and cut in half lengthwise. Scoop out the flesh. Chop flesh and mix with spinach and bell pepper. Season to taste and fill the eggplant halves. Bake in the oven.

Shortly before the eggplants are done put an egg on top of each half and finish baking.

Season turkey medallions with coarse pepper and roast in the oven for about 15 minutes. Make sure that they do not dry out. If necessary, remove earlier from the oven or put in 10 minutes later on a baking tray. Garnish at the end with creamy goat's cheese.

Vegetarians can leave out the meat and eat 2 boats instead.

For those who are not on the diet: a delicious low-carb dinner – with no regrets.

Steak with Barbecue Sauce

Nutritional values

Approx. total
470 kcal
(1969 kJ)
0.39 oz F
0.92 oz C
2.12 oz P

Ingredients:

1	Steak
4 oz	Tomato paste
3 tbsp	Cider vinegar
3 tbsp	Lemon juice
2-3 dashes	Tabasco
1	Onion, finely chopped
2 cloves	Garlic, finely chopped
1 pinch	Chilli powder to taste
1/2 tsp	Soy sauce
1 tsp	Parsley, finely chopped
	Cayenne pepper, salt and pepper, liquid stevia, xylitol or Sukrin.

Preparation:

Mix and stir all ingredients in a small pot and bring to the boil. If necessary add some water. Fry the steak in a non-stick pan or grill it. Done!

STABILIZATION AND TEST PHASE

Lamb´s Lettuce with Diced Red Beets and Chicken Breast

Ingredients:

2	Red beets
2	Small onions
1 bowl	Lamb´s lettuce
5 oz	Chicken breast
1-1/3 Cups	Vegetable stock without MSG
1 clove	Garlic, chopped
1	Bay leaf
	Sea salt, black pepper
	Balsamic vinegar
1	Lemon

Nutritional values

Approx. total
357 kcal
(1490 kJ)
0.07 oz F
1.23 oz C
1.52 oz P

Preparation:

Wash and dice the beets. Peel and dice the onions. Cook both in the vegetable stock together with the bay leaf on medium heat until the beets are cooked through. Take off the heat and set aside to cool. Add the balsamic vinegar to the warm beets. Season to taste with salt, pepper and lemon juice. Cut the chicken breast into 2-inch strips and fry in a non-stick pan. Add chopped garlic and season to taste with salt and pepper.

Wash the lamb's lettuce and arrange on a platter, season to taste with salt, pepper and balsamic vinegar. Add beets and season to taste. Place warm chicken breast on the salad and drizzle with lemon juice.

Mixed Salad with Beef Tenderloin

Ingredients:

1	Beef Tenderloin
	Salt, pepper
1 portion	Mixed salad leaves of your choice
1/2	Blood orange
	Balsamic vinegar
	Goat's cheese

Nutritional values

Approx. total
506 kcal
(2468 kJ)
0.59 oz F
0.74 oz C
2.22 oz P

Preparation:

Wash the salad, tear into small pieces and arrange on a platter. Cut the tenderloin into strips and fry quickly on a high heat. Cook until the meat is still pink (medium). Season to taste and place on top of the salad.

Squeeze the blood orange and add a dash of balsamic vinegar. Season to taste with salt and pepper. Mix well and drizzle over the salad. If desired sprinkle a few pieces of goat's cheese on top.

For those who are not on the diet: add a dash of walnut oil and a few walnuts.

STABILIZATION AND TEST PHASE

Chicken Escalopes Stuffed with Spinach and Peppers and Celery Root Purée

Nutritional values

Approx. total		
715	kcal	
(2994	kJ)	
0.25 oz	F	
1.52 oz	C	
4.13 oz	P	

Ingredients:

7 oz	Spinach
7 oz	Bell peppers
4	Chicken escalopes
14 oz	Fresh tomatoes
	Rosemary
7 oz	Celery root
7 oz	Parsnips
	Salt, pepper, garlic

Preparation:

Briefly sauté the spinach and peppers. Slice the chicken breast into escalopes and pound flat. Spread with the spinach and pepper mixture and roll up. Tie with string or secure with a tooth pick and brown quickly in a pan.

Place the escalopes in a casserole dish. Add fresh tomatoes and rosemary. Bake for 15 min in the oven.

Put the peeled and cubed celery root in another pot with some water. Add parsnips and seasonings and bring to a boil. As soon as the vegetables are cooked, remove from the water (the water can be used later for a delicious soup)

Put the cooked vegetables into a food processor and purée. Season with salt, pepper, garlic and other spices.

The purée tastes delicious with a little butter.

For those who are not on the diet: this is a fantastic low-carb dinner.

Cauliflower Pizza
(Recipe for 2 round 11 inch pizzas)

Nutritional values

Approx. total		
1936	kcal	
(8101	kJ)	
4.40 oz	F	
2.50 oz	C	
4.30 oz	P	

Ingredients:

1	Onion
2 tbsp	Olive oil
1 can	Chopped tomatoes (14 oz)
	Salt, pepper, pizza spices without MSG
2lb	Cauliflower
3-4	Tomatoes
1-2	Peppers
9 oz	Mozzarella
7 oz	Gouda cheese, grated
	Basil

Preparation:

Heat olive oil in a pan and fry the onions. Add the chopped tomatoes, bring to the boil and simmer for 5 minutes, stirring continuously. Season with salt, pepper and pizza spices.

Wash the cauliflower, cut florets and blanch for 4 minutes in salted boiling water. Drain and rinse with cold water. Cut the fresh tomatoes and the mozzarella into slices. Now cut the peppers into slices.

For the pizza crust, coarsely chop the cauliflower in a food processor and stir in the grated Gouda. Spread on two silicone pizza baking sheets and bake in a pre-heated fan oven at 400° F.

Remove from the oven and spread the tomato sauce over the pizza crust and cover with the slices of tomato, mozzarella and pepper.

Bake in a hot oven for about 15 min. When ready, garnish with finely chopped basil.

STABILIZATION AND TEST PHASE

Broccoli Salmon Casserole

Nutritional values

Approx. total:
884 kcal
(3704 kJ)
1.73 oz F
0.53 oz C
3.20 oz P

Ingredients:

9 oz	Salmon
1 lb	Broccoli
	Salt, pepper, paprika
	Emmenthal and Parmesan cheese to taste

Preparation:

Place the salmon in a casserole dish. Add the broccoli and season to taste.

Sprinkle the grated cheese over the salmon and the broccoli, as desired.

Bake in a fan oven at 350° F for 25-35 minutes until the cheese is golden brown.

Chilli con Carne

Nutritional values

Approx. total:
1333 kcal
(5587 kJ)
1.52 oz F
2.78 oz C
5.57 oz P

Ingredients:

14 oz	Stewing beef
1-2	Onions
2 oz	Pinto beans
2 oz	Corn
2-2/3 cups	Beef stock
1 lb can	Tomatoes
2	Chilli peppers
7 oz	Low-fat quark
1 bunch	Swiss chard
1 tsp each	Paprika, cumin, coriander seeds

Preparation:

Brown the chopped meat in a large pot. Chop the onions, chilli peppers and Swiss chard and add to the meat. Add pinto beans and corn and cook for approximately 2 hours until the meat is tender and falls apart.

Season the chilli con carne with spices, salt and pepper.

Garnish with curd cheese.

STABILIZATION AND TEST PHASE

Fish Soup

Ingredients:

10-1/2 oz	Mixed fish or seafood of your choice, cut into large cubes
1 stalk	Lemon grass, finely sliced
1	Fennel bulb, finely sliced
2 cups	Chinese cabbage, finely sliced
2	Spring onions, finely sliced
1 clove	Garlic, finely chopped
1 tbsp	Soy sauce
1/4 inch	Ginger root, finely chopped
1/2 tsp	Sambal Olek
	Saffron threads or powder
1 dash	Lemon juice
2-2/3 cups	Vegetable stock (without MSG)
	Fresh coriander, salt and pepper

Nutritional values

Approx. total:
- 381 kcal
- (1590 kJ)
- 0.18 oz F
- 0.59 oz C
- 2.19 oz P

Preparation:

Bring the stock to a boil and add all the ingredients, except for the fish and coriander, and simmer for 5 minutes. Then add the fish and simmer for a further 5 minutes. Season with salt and pepper.

Wash the coriander, pat dry and then tear into small pieces. Before serving, sprinkle over the soup.

Baked asparagus with leeks and turkey breast

Ingredients:

1 lb	Fresh asparagus
9 oz	Turkey breast, smoked
7 oz	Cottage cheese
1/2	Leek
1	Egg
2 oz	Parmesan, freshly grated

Nutritional values

Approx. total:
- 900 kcal
- (3757 kJ)
- 1.27 oz F
- 0.67 oz C
- 4.30 oz P

Preparation:

Peel the asparagus and finely slice the washed leek. Mix the cottage cheese with the egg. Season with salt and pepper.

Place all the ingredients in a casserole dish, sprinkle with the freshly grated Parmesan and bake for 30 min at 300° F in a fan oven.

STABILIZATION AND TEST PHASE

Stuffed Chicken Breast

Nutritional values
Approx. total:
  1480 kcal
 (6187 kJ)
  1.41 oz F
  0.74 oz C
  9.14 oz P

Ingredients:

9 oz	Ricotta
3 sprigs	Tarragon
3 sprigs	Parsley
	Salt, pepper
6	Chicken breasts (about 5-1/2 oz)
1/2	Lemon
1 tbsp	Honey
	Rapeseed oil for grilling

Preparation:

Drain the ricotta in a fine sieve for at least 4 hours. Finely chop the herbs. Mix with the drained ricotta, season with salt and pepper.

Wash the chicken breasts and pat dry. Make an incision at the upper end of the chicken breasts to form a pocket. Fill a pastry bag with the ricotta mixture and stuff each chicken breast. Secure with 2 toothpicks.

Place the chicken in a casserole dish. Mix 1 tbsp of lemon juice with the honey.

Coat the chicken breasts in the marinade, cover and refrigerate for 2 hours. Remove chicken from the marinade and drain.

Place the chicken breasts on a lightly oiled grill or under the grill in a pre-heated oven. Turn several times for 12 minutes. Season with salt and pepper and serve immediately.

Stuffed Mozzarella

Nutritional values
Approx. total:
  782 kcal
 (2369 kJ)
  2.12 oz F
  0.32 oz C
  2.82 oz P

Ingredients:

2 balls	Mozzarella (about 4-1/2 oz)
1 1/2 bunches	Parsley
1	Tomato
1	Spring onion
1 tbsp	Vinegar
1 tbsp	Oil
	Salt, pepper

Preparation:

Scoop out the inside of the mozzarella balls and cut into dice. Finely chop the parsley. Halve the tomato and cut into small dice. Finely slice the spring onion.

Mix vinegar, salt and pepper and pour on to the tomato-mozzarella-mixture. Stuff the mozzarella boats and serve the rest in a separate bowl.

STABILIZATION AND TEST PHASE

Stuffed Turkey Rolls

Nutritional values

Approx. total:
1200 kcal
(5020 kJ)
2.89 oz F
1.38 oz C
2.65 oz P

Ingredients:

1 oz	Walnuts
7 oz	Celery root
	Salt
7 oz	Apples
3 tbsp	Natural yoghurt
	Pepper
1 tbsp	Worcestershire sauce
	Tabasco
7 oz	(approx. 8 slices) smoked turkey breast
1 small	Lemon
7 oz	Avocado, ripe
1 tbsp	Olive oil

Preparation:

Coarsely chop the walnuts and toast briefly in a pan without oil. Peel and wash the celery root and cut into thin slices. Blanch for 1 minute in boiling salted water.

Drain and rinse in cold water. Core the apple and cut into thin slices.

Mix the celery root, apple, walnuts and yoghurt in a bowl. Season with salt, pepper, Worcestershire sauce and Tabasco. Place some celery root salad on each turkey piece and roll. Secure with a toothpick. Squeeze the lemon.

Halve the avocado, remove the stone and loosen the flesh from the peel. Cut into slices and arrange on a platter.

Season with salt, pepper and 1-2 tbsp of lemon juice. Drizzle with oil. Place the turkey rolls on top and serve.

STABILIZATION AND TEST PHASE

Salad of Green Beans and Feta Cheese

Nutritional values

Approx. total:
831 kcal
(3488 kJ)
2.19 oz F
0.99 oz C
1.38 oz P

Ingredients

I lb	Green beans
5-1/2 oz	Cherry tomatoes
1 small	Onion (approx. 2 oz)
5-1/2 oz	Feta cheese
4 tbsp	Balsamic vinegar, white
3 tbsp	Olive oil
	Salt & pepper

Preparation:

Wash the beans and cook for 8-10 minutes in boiling salted water until "al dente". Drain and rinse in cold water. Pat dry and set aside to cool.

In the meantime, cut the cherry tomatoes into quarters. Then halve them again. Peel the onion and cut into thin rings.

For the salad dressing: mix the onions, salt, pepper and oil. Gently toss the beans and tomatoes in the dressing. Arrange on two plates and crumble the feta cheese over the two salads.

TIP:

You can prepare this salad a few hours before serving. Simply cover and set aside in a cool place and allow to marinate. However, only crumble the feta cheese over the salad just before serving.

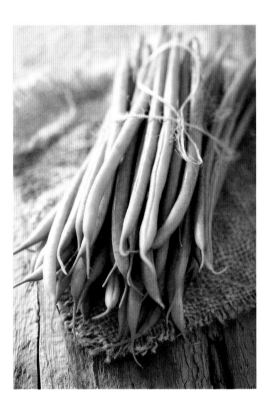

STABILIZATION AND TEST PHASE

Rolled Roast Meat Loaf

Nutritional values

Approx. total:
2074 kcal
(8701 kJ)
2.58 oz F
0.74 oz C
11.57 oz P

Ingredients:

2lbs	Lean hamburger
4 oz	Onion
7 oz	Cottage cheese
7 oz	Turkey breast slices, smoked
5 oz	Frozen spinach
3	Eggs
7 oz	Crushed tomatoes
2 tbsp	Parsley, chopped
	Pepper, cumin

Preparation:

Hard boil the eggs, cool under running cold water and peel. Finely chop the onion. Keep 1/4 for the tomato sauce.

Mix hamburger, cottage cheese, the remaining chopped onions, pepper, cumin and parsley.

Tear off a 20 inch piece of aluminum foil. With the matt side up, place the smoked turkey breast slices on it, overlapping each slice. Now spread half an inch of the hamburger over the turkey. Place the cooked eggs covered with the spinach at one end.

Starting from the end with the eggs and spinach, use the aluminum foil like filo pastry to make a meat roll. The eggs should now be in the middle of the loaf.

Put the rolled loaf in a casserole dish with a little water in the bottom and cover with a lid or foil. Cook for 30 minutes at 400° F. Remove the lid and brown for last 10 minutes.

During cooking you can prepare the sauce. Sweat the onions in a pan with some oil until soft then add the crushed tomatoes. Let the sauce simmer for 10 minutes. Season with salt and pepper.

Enjoy the sliced roast with the sauce.

TIP:

This roast is ideal to put portion-size slices in the freezer.

STABILIZATION AND TEST PHASE

Meat Pie

Nutritional values

Approx. total:
  3190 kcal
(13383 kJ)
6.24 oz F
1.62 oz C
12.31 oz P

Ingredients:

2 lbs	Lean hamburger
7 oz	Feta
2	Eggs
1-2	Leeks
2	Bell peppers
1-2	Onions
	Salt, pepper
4-5	Tomatoes
5 oz	Grated cheese

Preparation:

Mix together the hamburger, cubed feta and eggs. Cut the bell peppers into cubes, chop the onions, cut the leeks into rings or finely chop in an electric food processor. Mix everything together and season with salt and pepper. Place everything in a casserole dish and cover with tomato slices and grated cheese.

Chicken kebabs with Peanut Sauce

Nutritional values

Approx. total:
  1221 kcal
(5110 kJ)
2.61 oz F
0.71 oz C
4.20 oz P

Ingredients:

14 oz	Chicken breasts
7 oz	Coconut milk, unsweetened
2 tbsp	Peanut butter
2 tbsp	Peanuts, roasted and salted
1 tbsp	Curry paste
1 tbsp	Soy sauce
1	Lemon

Preparation:

For the sauce: on a medium heat, whisk the coconut milk with the peanut butter. Then add the curry paste, soy sauce and lemon juice to taste. Add the peanuts.

Cut the chicken breasts into equal cubes and thread on to wooden skewers.

Sear quickly for 5 minutes on both sides.

Arrange skewers and peanut sauce on a platter.

STABILIZATION AND TEST PHASE

Hamburgers

Nutritional values

Approx. total:
  1519 kcal
  (6370 kJ)
  3.45 oz F
  0.42 oz C
  5.22 oz P

Ingredients:

1lb	lean hamburger
4 oz	Ground flaxseed
2	Eggs
2 tbsp	Butter, melted
1 tbsp	Baking powder
2 tbsp	Tomato paste or sugar-free ketchup
1/2	Onion
1	Tomato

Preparation:

Pre-heat the oven to 400° F. Mix the flaxseed, eggs, butter and baking powder.

Divide the mixture in half and put hamburger size portions on a baking tray lined with waxed paper and bake in the oven for approximately 20 minutes until the burger buns are firm and slightly crunchy.

Season the hamburger meat and form into 2 patties. Fry in a pan until done. Slice the burger buns and spread tomato paste or sugar-free ketchup on them. Add the meat, lettuce, tomato and onion rings.

Harzer Cheese Salad

Nutritional values

Approx. total:
  718 kcal
  (2973 kJ)
  0.92 oz F
  1.99 oz C
  3.14 oz P

Ingredients:

2/3 Cup	Naturally cloudy apple juice
1 tsp	Mustard seeds
1 tsp	Xylitol or Sukrin
2 tbsp	Cider vinegar
1/2 tsp	Salt
	Pepper
2 tbsp	Cold-pressed rapeseed oil
7 oz	Radish
2 small	Onions, red
10 – 1/2 oz	Harzer cheese or another low fat cheese
1 bunch	Chives
	Lettuce, as much as you like

Preparation:

Place the apple juice, mustard seeds, xylitol or sukrin, vinegar and salt in a pot and bring to a boil. Cook on a high heat until reduced by half. Season with pepper, mix in the oil with a whisk and allow to cool. Peel and finely slice the radish. Peel the onion and slice into thin rings (or cut finely with a mandolin).

Cut the cheese into slices and put in a bowl together with the radish and onions. Pour the dressing over it, toss and marinate for 10 minutes.

STABILIZATION AND TEST PHASE

Chicken Breast with Peanut Sauce

Ingredients:

1-1/4 lbs	Chicken breasts
4 tbsp	Peanut oil
14 oz	Chinese cabbage
7 oz	Soybean sprouts
7 oz	Zucchini
2 tsp	Ground ginger
2 tsp	Curry powder
1 tsp	Cumin
4 tbsp	Soy sauce
3/4 oz	Peanut mousse

Nutritional values

Approx. total:
1403 kcal
(5862 kJ)
2.19 oz F
1.23 oz C
6.14 oz P

Preparation:

Cut the chicken breasts, zucchini and Chinese cabbage into small cubes. Heat oil in a pan or wok and fry the chicken breasts.

Now add the spices and vegetables and stir fry for 4 minutes.

Whisk the soy sauce and the peanut mousse with a fork and pour over the meat and vegetables. Mix well.

Salmon Spinach Roll

Ingredients:

4	Eggs
1 package	Smoked salmon
1 pack	age Spinach, frozen (or fresh)
7 oz	Cream cheese

Nutritional values

Approx. total:
1397 kcal
(5856 kJ)
3.70 oz F
0.32 oz C
3.70 oz P

Preparation:

Separate the eggs and beat the egg whites until stiff.

Mix the yolk with the spinach, season and carefully mix together.

Spread the spinach mixture on a baking tray and bake for 10-12 min. at 350° F in a fan oven. Next spread the cream cheese on the spinach crust and top with the salmon. Roll up and cut into slices.

Leek Soup with Ground Beef

Nutritional values

Approx. total:
1529 kcal
(6392 kJ)
2.96 oz F
1.27 oz C
5.33 oz P

Ingredients:

1 lb	Lean hamburger
2 lbs	Leeks
1 package	Soft cheese
	Salt, pepper
	Water or milk

Preparation:

Fry the meat and season with salt and pepper. Cut the leeks into fine slices and add to the hamburger meat a little at a time.

Add a little water or milk and simmer. Next add the soft cheese and allow to melt. Correct the seasoning. Enjoy!

Low Carb Lasagne

Nutritional values

Approx. total:
1194 kcal
(5015 kJ)
1.73 oz F
0.88 oz C
5.68 oz P

Ingredients:

For the "pasta dough":

1	Egg
3/4 Cup + 1 tbsp	Soy flour or flax seed meal
1 oz	Locust bean gum powder
1/2-3/4 Cup	Water
2-3 pinches	Salt

For the Sauce:

1 lb	Lean hamburger
1-2	Onions
	Salt, pepper
18 oz	Crushed tomatoes

Preparation:

Put the egg, flax seed meal or soy flour, salt, locust bean gum powder and 1/2 Cup water in a bowl and knead well either by hand or with a food processor using the dough hook attachment. If the dough is too crumbly, simply add more water.

Fry the onions. Season the hamburger and add to the onions. Add crushed tomatoes and season to taste.

Put one layer of the dough in a casserole dish and spread with the sauce. Repeat until the dish is full. If you like, garnish with grated cheese.

Bake in a fan oven at 400° F until slightly browned.

STABILIZATION AND TEST PHASE

Low Carb Pizza

Ingredients:

3	Eggs
1 tbsp	Warm water
	Salt, pepper, curry
5 oz	Ground almonds
	Pizza herbs
14 oz	Canned tomatoes
7 oz	Cheese

Nutritional values

Approx. total:
1773	kcal
(7428	kJ)
5.15 oz	F
0.74 oz	C
3.39 oz	P

Preparation:

Beat the eggs until foamy and add the spices. Next add the ground almonds. Spread the mixture evenly in a 9 x 11 inch silicone pan or a square baking pan lined with waxed paper.

First bake the pizza crust for 10-15 minutes in a fan oven at 400° F. Then top with the tomatoes, pizza herbs and cheese. Bake for about another 20 minutes at 400° F until the cheese is golden brown.

TIP:

The crust can be topped with other vegetables such as peppers, mushrooms etc.

Marinated Mozzarella

Ingredients:

1/2	Lime
1 oz	Green olives (pitted)
2 oz	Sun dried tomatoes
2 tbsp	Olive oil
1 small	Dried chilli pepper
9 oz	Mozzarella
	Black pepper
	Rosemary to garnish

Nutritional values

Approx. total:
1001	kcal
(4181	kJ)
2.9 oz	F
0.53 oz	C
1.87 oz	P

Preparation:

In a bowl, add 1 tbsp of the lime juice to the chopped olives, sun dried tomatoes and olive oil. Add chopped chilli pepper.

Drain the mozzarella and cut into small pieces. Arrange on a platter and season with the black pepper. Pour the dressing over it and marinate for 15 minutes at room temperature. Garnish with rosemary.

STABILIZATION AND TEST PHASE

Marinated Tuna

Ingredients:

1	Dried chilli pepper
	Paprika powder, hot
2 tbsp	Olive oil
4	Tuna steaks (about 6 oz)
2 red	Onions
2 oz	Capers
2 oz	Sun dried tomatoes in oil
1 tbsp	Balsamic vinegar
	Salt, pepper
3 sprigs	Oregano

Nutritional values

Approx. total:
1734	kcal	
(7303	kJ)	
4.48 oz	F	
0.56 oz	C	
4.80 oz	P	

Preparation:

Crumble the chilli pepper and mix with the paprika. Add the olive oil.

Wash the tuna, pat dry and toss in the chilli oil. Set aside in a cool place and the flavors to develop.

Peel and dice the onions. Drain and coarsely chop the capers. Drain the tomatoes, set 2 tbsp of the oil aside then chop them.

Combine the onion cubes, capers and tomatoes in a bowl with the vinegar and tomato oil. Season with salt and pepper. Coarsely chop the oregano leaves and add to the dressing.

Take the tuna from the chilli oil. Grill on a very hot grill for 1 minute on each side so that the fish remains medium rare. Next, roughly chop the tuna and mix with the remaining ingredients and marinate for another 15 min. Serve.

Mediterranean Baked Vegetables

Ingredients:

Mushrooms, zucchini, tomatoes, bell peppers (as many vegetables as you wish)
Olive oil
Fresh or dried rosemary

Preparation:

Slice the vegetables. Brush a baking tray with olive oil, spread with the vegetables and sprinkle with the rosemary. Roast at 400° F on the middle shelf of the oven for 35 minutes. Turn the vegetables once or twice while roasting.

TIP:

This goes well with grilled turkey breast, or 2-1/2 oz sour cream mixed with 3 tbsp milk, salt and pepper. The roasted vegetables can be combined with, for example, Brussels sprouts, kohlrabi, fennel and a little sheep's cheese.

STABILIZATION AND TEST PHASE

Mushrooms in Balsamic Vinegar

Ingredients:

1 lb	Assorted mushrooms
2 cloves	Garlic
2 sprigs	Parsley
2 tbsp	Olive oil
	Salt, pepper
3/4 Cup	Vegetable stock (without MSG)
3 tbsp	Balsamic vinegar

Nutritional values

Approx. total:
299 kcal
(1250 kJ)
0 oz F
0.42 oz C
0.53 oz P

Preparation:

Clean the mushrooms with a brush or paper towel and cut into uniform pieces.

Peel the garlic and chop finely.

Coarsely chop the parsley.

Heat the oil in a pan and sauté the garlic for 1 minute until golden brown.

Add the mushrooms and stir fry for 3-4 minutes. Season with salt and pepper.

Add the vegetable stock and chopped parsley. Let simmer for 1 minute.

Add the balsamic vinegar and simmer for 2-3 minutes. Set aside for 2 hours before serving.

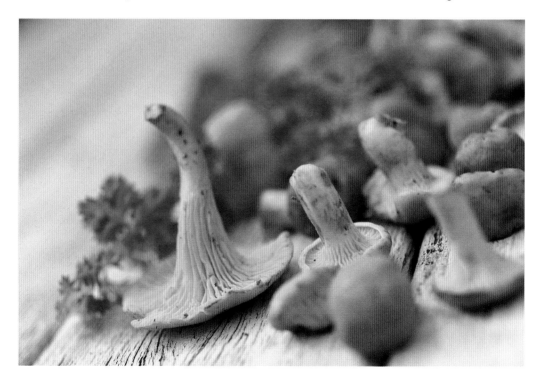

Pizza Meat Loaf

Ingredients:

4 oz	Sun dried tomatoes
2	Onions
2 lbs	Lean hamburger
1 tbsp	each thyme and parsley
	Mustard, medium
	Salt, pepper
2/3 Cup	Full fat plain yoghurt
1	Egg
2 tbsp	Oil
1 tsp	Xylitol or Sukrin
2 tbsp	Tomato paste
	Paprika powder, sweet
1 large can	Tomatoes (around 28 oz)
1-1/2 oz	Rocket
10 slices	Parma ham
	Plastic wrap
	Waxed paper

Nutritional values

Approx. total:
2846 kcal
(11920 kJ)
4.83 oz F
2.36 oz C
11.64 oz P

Preparation:

Finely chop the tomatoes and onions. In a bowl combine the hamburger meat, half the onions, herbs, mustard, 1-1/2 tsp salt, 1-1/2 tsp pepper, the yoghurt and the egg. Mix well in an electric food processor.

Drain the mozzarella and cut into cubes. Place the meat mixture on a piece of plastic wrap and press on to a flat plate (approx. 9 in x 9 in). Spread the mozzarella evenly over the meat, leaving a one inch border.

Using the plastic wrap, roll up the meat and form a loaf with your hands. Remove the plastic and score the surface several times with a knife. Place on a baking tray lined with waxed paper and cook in a pre-heated oven (325º F / fan: 300º F) for about an hour.

In the meantime, heat the oil for the sauce and sauté the rest of the onions. Add a little xylitol or sukrin, the tomato paste and simmer briefly. Season with the salt, pepper and paprika. Deglaze with the canned tomatoes. Bring to the boil and simmer for about 10 minutes. Correct the seasoning. Keep warm.

Wash the rocket and drain well. Quickly dry fry the ham and then remove. Next, take the meat out of the oven. Arrange on a platter together with the Parma ham and rocket. Serve with the sauce.

STABILIZATION AND TEST PHASE

Turkey Breast Greek style

Ingredients:

7 oz	Turkey breast
4 oz	Feta
7 oz	Sieved tomatoes (Passata)
1-2	Bell peppers
7 oz	Mushrooms
	Salt, pepper, chilli, herbes de Provence

Nutritional values

Approx. total:
624 kcal
(2616 kJ)
0.85 oz F
0.88 oz C
2.68 oz P

Preparation:

Season the turkey with salt, pepper and chilli and brown in a pan together with the mushrooms. Cut the feta into 1/2 inch cubes and cut the bell pepper into bite-size pieces. Place the turkey in a casserole dish, cover with the vegetables and feta. Correct the seasoning.

Bake at 400° F for about 30 min. Next, stir the sieved tomatoes into the pan juices, adding 3-4 tbsp water, if necessary. Make sure the sauce does not become too thin. Season with pepper and the herbes de Provence. Serve the turkey with the tomato sauce.

Radish Apple Salad

Ingredients:

1	White radish
1	Apple
1 tbsp	Mustard, sugar free
2 tbsp	Creamed horseradish
	A little whipping cream
2 oz	Walnuts

Nutritional values

Approx. total:
655 kcal
(2740 kJ)
1.80 oz F
1.31 oz C
0.42 oz P

Preparation:

Peel the radish and cut into thin slices. Cut the apple into small pieces then add the remaining ingredients and toss well. As easy as one-two-three!

STABILIZATION AND TEST PHASE

Rocket Salad with Poached Egg

Ingredients:

7 oz	Rocket
5 tbsp	Balsamic vinegar, white
2 tbsp	Olive oil
1	Egg
4 oz	Cooked ham
1 bunch	Chives

Nutritional values

Approx. total:
543	kcal	
(2263	kJ)	
1.20 oz	F	
0.56 oz	C	
1.55 oz	P	

Preparation:

Bring a little water to the boil. Add 2 tbsp Balsamic vinegar and break the egg into a cup and carefully pour into the boiling water. Poach for 5 minutes. Mix the remaining vinegar with the oil, salt and pepper. Slice the ham. Mix together the rocket, ham and dressing. Drain the poached egg and place on the salad. Garnish with some snipped chives.

Sweet and Sour Leek Salad with Yoghurt Sauce

Ingredients:

2	Leeks
1 cup	Celery (grated)
4	Hard boiled eggs
3	Apples (grated)
9 – 11 oz	Yoghurt
	Salt, pepper

Nutritional values

Approx. total:
986	kcal	
(4121	kJ)	
1.45 oz	F	
3.42 oz	C	
1.73 oz	P	

Preparation:

Halve the leeks lengthwise and rinse under running water and cut into thin slices.

Place in a bowl together with the grated celery.

Peel the eggs, slice them and add. Peel and core the apples, grate them and add to the other ingredients. Finally add the yoghurt and toss well.

Season with salt and pepper. Set aside and allow the flavors to develop.

TIP:

This salad is ideal as a takeaway.

STABILIZATION AND TEST PHASE

Ham and Asparagus Omelette

Nutritional values

Approx. total:
676 kcal
(2833 kJ)
1.45 oz F
0.21 oz C
2.50 oz P

Ingredients:

2-1/2 oz	Smoked chicken breast or lean ham
1 tsp	Olive oil
6	Egg whites
4	Eggs
4 oz	Canned asparagus
	Pepper, freshly ground

Preparation:

Brush a non-stick pan with the olive oil. Quickly fry the smoked chicken breast or lean ham. With an electric mixer, whisk the eggs and egg whites until foamy. Season with pepper and pour over the meat.

Cut the asparagus into small pieces and spread over the eggs. Cook for 8 minutes on medium heat.

Spaghetti Carbonara

Nutritional values

Approx. total:
1400 kcal
(5861 kJ)
2.33 oz F
3 oz C
4 oz P

Ingredients:

6 oz	Soy noodles or low carb noodles
4 oz	Turkey breast, smoked and sliced
4 oz	Low fat cottage cheese
4 oz	Parmesan cheese, freshly grated
3	Eggs

Preparation:

Spread turkey breast slices evenly on a baking tray and bake at 300° F until crisp.

Boil the water for the pasta. Add a pinch of salt.

Beat the eggs in a heat resistant bowl and add the low fat cottage cheese and parmesan. Whisk together until smooth.

Cook the soy pasta or low carb pasta in boiling water.

Stir the carbonara sauce in a pot over the boiling water.

When al dente, drain the pasta and toss in the carbonara sauce. Season with salt and pepper.

Crumble the crisp turkey breast slices over the pasta carbonara and enjoy!

STABILIZATION AND TEST PHASE

Asparagus and Carrot-Salad

Nutritional values

Approx. total:
692	kcal
(2898	kJ)
1.70 oz	F
1.40 oz	C
0.88 oz	P

Ingredients:

9 oz	Fresh white asparagus
9 oz	Fresh green asparagus
	Salt
1 tbsp	Olive oil
2 tbsp	Sherry vinegar
	Juice of 1/2 lemon
1 tsp	Mustard
2 tbsp	Sunflower oil
1 oz	Pine nuts
1 handful	Salad, e.g. lamb's lettuce
1/2 bunch	Parsley
1/2 bunch	Chervil (if available)
	Pepper
14 oz	Carrots

Preparation:

Wash the asparagus. Peel the white asparagus. Cut the asparagus into pieces and fry in hot oil for 4-5 minutes. Season with salt and pepper.

Peel and cut the carrots into pieces. Blanch in salted water for 3 minutes. Keep 2 tbsp of the carrot water and mix with the lemon juice, sherry vinegar, pepper, oil and mustard to make a dressing.

Toast the pine nuts, wash the salad and pat dry. Chop the herbs and add to the salad.

Toss the salad with the dressing. Enjoy!

Tuna and Tomato Stir Fry

Nutritional values

Approx. total:
1034	kcal
(4350	kJ)
2.30 oz	F
0.95 oz	C
3.10 oz	P

Ingredients:

2 cans	Tuna
1 cup	Sieved tomatoes (passata)
2	Onions
1 cup	Cream
	Salt, pepper
	Italian herbs

Preparation:

Sweat the onions in the oil until soft. Add the tuna and fry. Add the sieved tomatoes and season with salt, pepper and Italian herbs. Add the cream and warm up briefly before serving.

STABILIZATION AND TEST PHASE

Tomato Camembert Omelette

Nutritional values

Approx. total
931 kcal
(3902 kJ)
2.12 oz F
0.46 oz C
2.89 oz P

Ingredients:

4 oz	Small white mushrooms
4 oz	Cherry tomatoes
4 oz	Turkey breast, smoked
3-4	Eggs
	Fresh parsley
1/2 Cup	Milk
	Salt, pepper
	Paprika powder, sweet
4-1/2 oz	Camembert

Preparation:

Cut the mushrooms and tomatoes into quarters. Cube the smoked turkey breast. Whisk the eggs with the milk and season with salt, pepper and sweet paprika. Add the chopped parsley.

Heat up the oil in a non-stick frying pan and fry the mushrooms. Add the tomatoes and turkey breast and fry briefly. Pour egg and milk mixture evenly over them. Cover the pan and let it stand for 15 minutes on a gentle heat.

5 minutes before serving, cut the Camembert into slices and spread over the omelette.

Tomato Mozzarella Omelette

Nutritional values

Approx. total
1173 kcal
(4920 kJ)
3.21 oz F
0.67 oz C
2.47 oz P

Ingredients:

4-1/2 oz	Mozzarella
4	Tomatoes (medium)
5	Eggs
5-6 tbsp	Milk
	Salt, pepper
1 tsp	Paprika, sweet
3 tbsp	Rapeseed or olive oil
2 tsp	Italian herbs, frozen

Preparation:

Cut the mozzarella into cubes and slice the tomatoes. Mix the eggs and milk and season well with the salt, pepper and paprika.

Heat up 2 tbsp oil in a non-stick pan. Place half the tomato slices in the pan and sprinkle 1 tsp of the frozen herbs over them. Then spread half the mozzarella cubes over. Next layer the remaining tomato slices, herbs and mozzarella.

Pour in the egg and milk mixture and let stand for 15 minutes. Slide the omelette on to a large flat plate. Heat up 1 tbsp oil in the pan and gently slide the omelette back into the pan upside down. Cook for another 5 minutes. This tastes great with low carb bread.

STABILIZATION AND TEST PHASE

Lemon Chicken

Ingredients:

1-1/4 lb	Whole chicken, organic
1 lb	Green beans
9 oz	Vine tomatoes
1	Unwaxed lemon
1 sprig	Rosemary, fresh
2 sprigs	Thyme, fresh
1 clove	Garlic
1 tsp	Salt
1 tsp	Freshly ground pepper

Nutritional values

Approx. total
1222 kcal
(5122 kJ)
2.12 oz F
1.13 oz C
4.73 oz P

Preparation:

Pre-heat the oven to 400° F.

Wash the chicken and cut along its back with a sharp knife or poultry shears. Place breast side up on a baking tray lined with waxed paper. Press down to flatten slightly.

Grate the lemon, squeeze half the lemon and chop the herbs.

Combine the lemon juice, grated lemon peel, herbs, salt/pepper and chopped garlic to make a marinade.

Spread the marinade under the skin of the chicken, taking care not to tear the skin. Roast for 30 minutes on the middle shelf of a pre-heated oven.

Pierce the tomatoes, top and tail the beans and place around the chicken.

Cook for a further 30 minutes and serve.

STABILIZATION AND TEST PHASE

Zucchini Carpaccio

Ingredients:

10-1/2 oz	Green zucchini
5 oz	Yellow zucchini
3 tbsp	Olive oil
	Salt, pepper
1 oz	Sun dried tomatoes in oil
1 oz	Pitted green olives
1/2 bunch	Basil
6 oz	Ricotta
1	Dried chilli
3/4 oz	Pine nuts
3/4 oz	Rocket

Nutritional values

Approx. total
935 kcal
(3920 kJ)
2.86 oz F
0.88 oz C
1.09 oz P

Preparation:

Cut off the ends of the zucchini and cut into thin slices or finely slice with a mandolin.

Place the zucchini slices on a baking tray, brush with a little of the olive oil and season with the salt and pepper. Place on the middle shelf of a 425° F pre-heated oven (fan oven 400° F) and roast for 8 minutes. Remove and set aside to cool.

Drain and finely chop the sun dried tomatoes. Finely chop the olives and basil.

In a bowl, combine the tomatoes, olives, basil and ricotta. Season with salt, pepper and crumbled chilli.

Toast the pine nuts in a pan. Prepare the rocket. Arrange the roasted zucchini slices on a plate. Using two wet spoons, place scoops of the ricotta mixture next to the zucchini. Garnish with the pine nuts and rocket.

STABILIZATION AND TEST PHASE

Zucchini Salad

Ingredients:

> Zucchini
> Balsamic vinegar
> Olive or coconut oil for frying
> Salt, pepper

Preparation:

Wash the zucchini and cut into small pieces. Next fry the zucchini in a pan brushed with oil and season with the vinegar, salt and pepper.

Set aside to allow the flavors to develop. Enjoy hot or cold. This salad is ideal for a takeaway. It also tastes good with cubes of feta or other cheese.

Onion Quiche

Nutritional values

Approx. total
3262 kcal
(13669 kJ)
6.35 oz F
2.82 oz C
11.18 oz P

Ingredients:

Pastry Dough:

6	Eggs
1 tsp	Baking powder
1 tsp	Salt
7 oz	Low fat Quark
2 oz	Flax seeds
1-2/3 Cups	Soy flour
2 oz	Sunflower seeds

Onion topping:

2	Eggs
1-3/4 lbs	Onions
14 oz	Smoked turkey breast
2 tsp	Oil
7 oz	Sour cream 10 % fat
7 oz	Low fat Quark
	A little cumin, if desired

Preparation:

With an electric mixer, beat the eggs and the quark until foamy. Next add the dry ingredients.

Line a baking tray with waxed paper and spread the dough evenly. Cube the turkey breast and fry in the oil with the onions and set aside. Spread the onion mixture over the pastry base. Mix the sour cream into the quark and eggs, season and pour over the onion mixture.

Bake for 25-30 minutes at 350° F.

STABILIZATION AND TEST PHASE

Spicy Strips of Beef Tenderloin with Zucchini Spaghetti

Ingredients:

5 oz	Beef tenderloin
4 oz	Onions
6 tbsp	Vegetable stock without MSG
1	Chilli pepper
3	Zucchini
9 oz	Tomatoes
	Fresh herbs (e.g. Parsley)
	Sea salt, black pepper, curry powder
1	Lemon

Nutritional values

Approx. total
433 kcal
(1823 kJ)
0.39 oz F
1.13 oz C
1.76 oz P

Preparation:

Peel and finely slice the onions. In a non-stick saucepan, sauté half the onions with a little oil. Cut the tomatoes into large dice, add to the onions and sauté for 5 minutes. Add the vegetable stock and season with salt and pepper. Make zucchini spaghetti using a vegetable spiral cutter and briefly blanch for 20 seconds in boiling vegetable stock. Remove immediately and drain. Finely chop the chilli pepper and add to the onions.

Cut the tenderloin into strips with a sharp knife and dry fry in a very hot non-stick pan. Add the chilli and onions immediately. Season with the salt, pepper and curry powder. Finely chop the herbs.

Arrange the spaghetti on a plate, spoon over the tomato sauce and place the tenderloin strips on top. (Remember that the heat from the chilli comes from the seeds). Drizzle with lemon juice.

King Prawns on rocket

Ingredients:

6	King prawns
5 oz	Rocket
4 tsp	Vegetable stock (without MSG)
1	Onion
1 clove	Garlic
1	Belgian Endive
	Sea salt, black pepper
1	Lemon
4 tsp	Cider vinegar
1/2	Orange

Nutritional values

Approx. total
283 kcal
(1180 kJ)
0.18 oz F
0.67 oz C
1.34 oz P

Preparation:

Wash and peel the king prawns and season with the lemon juice and salt. Peel and dice the onions and garlic. In a pan, dry fry the onion and garlic. Add the prawns. Break apart the leaves of the Belgian endive and rinse in lukewarm water. (This eliminates any bitterness).

Prepare the rocket. Add the vegetable stock to the prawns, simmer and drizzle with lemon juice. Arrange the Belgian endive on a platter, next add the rocket and season with orange juice, salt and pepper. Garnish with the prawns – done!

STABILIZATION AND TEST PHASE

BREAD AND BREAD ROLLS

Apple Protein Bread

Ingredients:

7 oz	Protein powder
7 oz	Apples or frozen red berries
7 oz	Low fat Quark
2	Eggs
1-1/2 tbsp	Baking powder
1/2 tsp	Salt
1 tsp	Xylitol or Sukrin
1/2 tsp	Cinnamon

Nutritional values

Approx. total
1263 kcal
(5333 kJ)
0.60 oz F
1.59 oz C
8.25 oz P

Preparation:

Pureé the peeled apples (or thawed berries) and mix with the other ingredients. Knead well and place in a silicone loaf pan.

Bake in a fan oven at 300° F for 30-40 minutes.

Low Carb Apple Bread

Ingredients:

6-1/2 oz	Almond flour or ground almonds
4 oz	Cream cheese
5	Eggs
2 tsp	Cinnamon
1 tsp	Baking powder
1-1/2	Apples, finely chopped
1/2 cup	Melted butter
	Xylitol or Sukrin

Nutritional values

Approx. total
2625 kcal
(10995 kJ)
8.15 oz F
2.05 oz C
3.07 oz P

Preparation:

First beat the melted butter with the cream cheese and eggs. Then add the rest of the ingredients. Lastly, fold in the apple pieces.

Place everything in a loaf pan and bake at 300° F for 45 minutes.

STABILIZATION AND TEST PHASE

Chia Crackers

Ingredients:

1/4 cup	Chia seeds
1/2 cup	Ground flax seeds
1 cup	Water
1 tsp	Salt
	Herbes de Provence

Nutritional values

Approx. total
386 kcal
(1617 kJ)
0.99 oz F
0.53 oz C
0.71 oz P

Preparation:

Mix Chia and flax seeds with water and set aside for about 20 minutes to swell.

Then mix in all the ingredients and form small flat crackers on a baking tray lined with waxed paper.

Bake the crackers for about 1 hour at 300° F. NOTE: Keep the oven door open slightly with a wooden spoon, or something similar, to allow any moisture to escape.

The baking time can vary, depending on the oven and how crisp you want the crackers.

Walnut Bread

Ingredients:

4 oz	Sesame seeds
4oz	Flax seeds
4 oz	Walnuts, whole
4 oz	Almonds, whole
4 oz	Pumpkin seeds
4 oz	Sunflower seeds
4 oz	Protein powder, unflavored
6	Eggs
10-1/2 oz	Low fat Quark
2 tsp	Salt

Nutritional values

Approx. total
4458 kcal
(18697 kJ)
11.78 oz F
2.33 oz C
10.76 oz P

Preparation:

Mix all ingredients together with an electric hand mixer and place in a silicone loaf pan.

Pre-heat oven to 300° F and bake for one hour.

STABILIZATION AND TEST PHASE

Protein Bread

Nutritional values

Ingredients:

10 1/2 oz	Quark
5	Eggs
2 oz	Wheat bran
4 oz	Ground almonds
4 oz	Psyllium husks (or flax seed, Chia seeds, whole or ground)
1-1/2 tbsp	Baking powder
	Salt

Approx. total
1832 kcal
(7677 kJ)
4.48 oz F
1.69 oz C
4.52 oz P

Preparation:

Beat the eggs with the quark. Next add all the other ingredients and knead with dough hook attachment. Then place in a loaf pan.

Bake bread for about one hour at 300º F.

Low Carb Soy Bread

Nutritional values

Ingredients:

8	Eggs
2 tsp	Baking Powder
2 tsp	Salt
10-1/2 oz	Low fat Quark
4 oz	Linseeds or linseed meal
1-3/4 Cups	Soy flour
4 oz	Sunflower seeds
	Butter to grease the loaf pan

Approx. total
2721 kcal
(11401 kJ)
6.60 oz F
1.13 oz C
8.15 oz P

Preparation:

Pre-heat the oven to 350º F

Combine all the dry ingredients and then add the eggs and low fat quark. Mix into a smooth dough.

Grease and line a loaf pan with waxed paper or use a silicone loaf pan. Place the dough into the loaf pan and bake for 45 minutes at 350º F.

TIP:

The bread can also be baked in a bread maker. When using a bread maker, put the eggs and low fat quark in first and then add the remaining ingredients. Select "normal whole meal bread" program, dark crust.

STABILIZATION AND TEST PHASE

Low Carb Sour Dough Bread (makes about 20 slices)

Nutritional values

Approx. total
   3123 kcal
(13074 kJ)
5.36 oz F
9.56 oz C
5.86 oz P

Ingredients Sour dough:

4 oz	Chickpea flour
7 tbsp	Cider or herbal vinegar, naturally cloudy
	Soda or sparkling water (medium carbonation)

Ingredients sour dough starter:

1 lb	Chickpea flour
3-1/3 Cups	Sparkling or soda water (medium carbonation)

Ingredients main dough:

2-1/2 oz	Chickpea flour
2 tsp	Salt
5 oz	Flax seeds
3/4 oz	Sesame seeds
1-1/2 oz	Chopped almonds
1/2 Cup	100 % natural carrot juice
2 tbsp	Olive oil
	Sparkling or soda water (medium carbonation)
	Oil to grease the loaf pan

Preparation:

Step 1 – Sour dough:

Stir the chickpea flour and vinegar together and place in a large screw-top jar (minimum 1 lb size). Add some soda or sparkling water to make a thick, sticky mass. Place in a cool oven at 120º F for 3 hours to prove.

Step 2 – Starter

Place sour dough in a glass bowl or Pyrex dish and mix with the chickpea flour and sparkling water. Cover the bowl with a lid or plate and allow to prove for about 8 hours (or overnight) in the oven at 120º F.

Step 3 – Main dough

Mix the starter with all the remaining ingredients. Add some sparkling water if necessary. Place dough in a loaf pan, greased with olive oil and lined with waxed paper. Let it prove again for at least 3 more hours at 120º F.

Step 4 – Bake

Brush the top of the dough with a little olive oil and place in a cold oven. Bake for 90 minutes at 300º F. Take out the bread. Remove from the pan, brush the sides of the loaf with olive oil and bake for a further 30 minutes. Set aside to cool.

STABILIZATION AND TEST PHASE

Low Carb Bread with Almonds and Linseeds

Ingredients:

13 oz	Low fat Quark
10	Eggs
4-1/2 oz	Ground almonds
4-1/2 oz	Ground linseeds or partially hydrogenated linseed flour
3 oz	Wheat bran
2-1/2 tbsp	Soy flour
2-1/2 tbsp	Baking powder
1-1/2 tsp	Salt
2-1/2 tbsp	Sunflower seeds

Nutritional values

Approx. total
2844 kcal
(11922 kJ)
7.09 oz F
1.80 oz C
7.51 oz P

Preparation:

Mix the eggs, quark and remaining ingredients in an automatic bread maker. Since the dough contains many seeds and nuts, it may stick to the bowl of the bread maker. Scrape off with a spatula while the bowl is turning to ensure the dough is mixed evenly.

Select "normal whole meal bread" programme, dark crust.

TIP:

Bread can also be baked in a loaf pan at 300° F for 40 minutes. Pre-heat a fan oven to 300° F and maintain that temperature for 15 minutes before placing the bread in the oven. The dough can also be put in silicone muffin cups to make rolls.

Low Carb Bread Rolls

Ingredients: (for 8 rolls)

4	Eggs, salt
1/2 tsp	Lemon juice
4 oz	Wheat bran
4 oz	Ground flax seeds
4 oz	Protein powder, unflavored
2 tsp	Baking powder
1lb	Low fat Quark

Nutritional values

Approx. total
1695 kcal
(6643 kJ)
2.26 oz F
1.55 oz C
8.29 oz P

Preparation:

Separate the eggs. Add a pinch of salt and lemon juice to the egg whites and beat until stiff. Mix wheat bran, flax seed, protein powder, baking powder and 1 tsp salt. Beat egg yolks and quark until creamy. On a low speed, add the dry ingredients. Fold in the beaten egg whites. Leave the dough to prove for 10 minutes.

Pre-heat the oven to 325° F. Line a baking tray with waxed paper. Form 8 bread rolls. Cut a cross into the top. Bake on the middle shelf for 25-30 minutes.

STABILIZATION AND TEST PHASE

Low Carb Yeast Bread Rolls/Pizza Base

Ingredients:

1-3/4 Cups	Oat bran
2-1/2 oz	Gluten
1/2-1 tsp	Salt
1/4 tsp	Sugar
3/4 Cup	Lukewarm water
1/2 cube	Fresh yeast or 1 sachet instant yeast
2 oz	Low Fat Quark (room temperature)
1 tsp	Rapeseed oil

Nutritional values

Approx. total
1008 kcal
(4220 kJ)
0.78 oz F
3.35 oz C
3.35 oz P

Preparation:

Thoroughly mix the dry ingredients together. Add the remaining ingredients and knead for 5 minutes. Allow to prove for 40 minutes in a warm spot.

Form 6-8 rolls and place on a baking tray lined with waxed paper. Allow to prove for a further 20 minutes.

Bake in a fan oven for 25-30 minutes at 350° F.

TIP:

This type of dough is ideal for a pizza base or pizza spirals. Just incorporate some pizza spices into the dough. It can also be used for sweet things. Just add a pinch of salt and sweeten with xylitol, Sukrin or liquid stevia.

You can make a delicious apple dish if you roll the sweet dough into a rectangular silicone baking pan and add the following topping:

1-1/4 lbs finely chopped apples, 9 oz quark, 1 tsp cinnamon and 1 oz vanilla or coconut flavored protein powder. Bake at 350° F for 25-30 minutes in a fan oven.

STABILIZATION AND TEST PHASE

Low Carb "Oopsie" Bread

Nutritional values

Approx. total
620 kcal
(2598 kJ)
1.83 oz F
0.21 oz C
1.20 oz P

Ingredients:

3	Eggs
1 pinch	Salt
1 tsp	Baking powder
4 oz	Cream cheese
	Nuts, seeds (optional)

Preparation:

Separate the eggs. Next beat the whites with a hand mixer to the stiff peak stage. The stiffer the whites, the better the "oopsies" will turn out.

In another bowl, beat the yolks with the cream cheese. Gently fold in the egg whites.

Place the "oopsies" on a baking tray lined with waxed paper.

Bake at 300° F for 25-30 minutes. Done!

If you like, you can put all kinds of nuts, herbs or garlic powder into the "oopsie" dough.

Delicious with quark and watercress.

If you like them sweet just add a little cinnamon, xylitol, Sukrin or stevia powder.

TIP:

The "oopsies" make ideal hamburger buns.

Just use 2 "oopsies" and spread with tomato paste or sugar-free ketchup then layer on cucumber slices, tomato, a hamburger patty (made from lean ground beef) and cheese.

STABILIZATION AND TEST PHASE

Macadamia Bread

Nutritional values

Approx. total
1353 kcal
(5668 kJ)
3.70 oz F
0.35 oz C
4.27 oz P

Ingredients:

4	Eggs
10-1/2 oz	Macadamia nut flour
1-1/2 tbsp	Baking powder (with saffron)

Preparation:

In an electric food processor with the dough hook attachment, mix the eggs, macadamia nut flour and baking powder (saffron). Bake for 30 min. at 400° F.

And the macadamia bread is done!

Almond Bread / Almond Bread Rolls

Nutritional values

Approx. total
8260 kcal
(34594 kJ)
26.91 oz F
3.17 oz C
10.08 oz P

Ingredients:

6	Eggs
7 oz	Yoghurt
4 oz	Melted butter
2 tsp	Baking powder
2 tsp	Salt
1-3/4 lb	Ground almonds
7 oz	Sunflower seeds
7 oz	Sesame seeds

Preparation:

Beat the eggs and yoghurt until creamy and add the remaining ingredients. Spoon into silicone muffin cups or a silicone baking pan and bake for 40 minutes at 300 – 325° F.

TIP:

Instead of the ground almonds you can also use almond flour or all kinds of other nut flours.

STABILIZATION AND TEST PHASE

Soy Bread Rolls

Nutritional values

Approx. total
1674 kcal
(6769 kJ)
2.36 oz F
0.53 oz C
8.92 oz P

Ingredients:

7 oz	Soy flour or soy meal
5 oz	Gluten
2 oz	Protein powder, unflavored
6-1/2 tbsp	lukewarm water
1/2 tsp	Sugar
1/2 cube	fresh yeast
1 heaped tsp	Salt
2 tbsp	Rapeseed oil
1-1/2 Cups	lukewarm water

Preparation:

In a bowl, combine the soy flour or soy meal, gluten and unflavored protein powder and make a well.

Dissolve the sugar and yeast in the 6-1/2 tbsp lukewarm water and pour into the well. Cover with a cloth and set aside.

After 30 minutes, add the salt, rapeseed oil and 1-1/2 cups lukewarm water. Mix with a dough hook attachment until the dough can be easily removed from the bowl. Next, knead well. (You may want to dust your work surface with a little gluten).

Place the dough back in a bowl and cover with a damp cloth. Allow to prove for about 1 hour in a warm spot.

Next form rolls and place on a baking tray lined with waxed paper, score the tops and allow to rise for 15 minutes.

Bake in a pre-heated oven at 325° F for about 20 minutes.

TIP:

This kind of dough can be used also as pizza base or for sweet buns. (Simply sweeten with xylitol or Sukrin) or, for sweet pastries, with poppy seeds or nuts. There are no limits to your low carb imagination!

It is also much easier if made with a bread maker. In order to get a smooth dough simply put the liquid ingredients in first and then add the rest.

STABILIZATION AND TEST PHASE

Walnut Bread

Ingredients:

4 oz	Sesame seeds
4 oz	Flax seeds
4 oz	Walnuts whole
4 oz	Almonds whole
4 oz	Pumpkin seeds
4 oz	Sunflower seeds
1	Egg
6-1/2 tbsp	Olive or rapeseed oil
2 tsp	Salt

Nutritional values

Approx. total
4631 kcal
(19394 kJ)
15.03 oz F
1.87 oz C
5.64 oz P

Preparation:

Mix all the ingredients with a hand mixer and turn into a loaf pan.

Bake for 60 minutes at 300 to 325° F.

CAKES

Cheesecake

Ingredients:

5	Eggs
1 lb	Low fat Quark
	Stevia or xylitol or Sukrin
1 sachet	Vanilla pudding powder
	Vanilla, ground
1 tsp	Rapeseed or coconut oil

Nutritional values

Approx. total
1076 kcal
(4501 kJ)
1.59 oz F
2.12 oz C
3.84 oz P

Preparation:

Separate the eggs. Beat the egg whites until stiff. In a separate bowl, beat the yolks with the low fat quark until creamy and incorporate the remaining ingredients.

Lastly, fold in the egg whites and spoon into a silicone baking pan.

Bake at 300 to 325° F for 50 minutes.

Coconut Apple Muffins

	Nutritional values
	Approx. total
	3098 kcal
	(12973 kJ)
	8.08 oz F
	3.25 oz C
	5.89 oz P

Ingredients:

4 oz	Ground almonds
4 oz	Ground hazelnuts
4 oz	protein powder vanilla or coconut
1-1/2 tbsp	Baking powder
4 oz	Grated coconut
7 oz	Ricotta or low fat Quark
9 oz	Buttermilk
3	Eggs
2	Apples

Preparation:

Mix the ground almonds and hazelnuts, protein powder and grated coconut. With a hand mixer, beat the eggs, ricotta and buttermilk until smooth. Next, stir in the dry ingredients.

With an electric food processor, finely chop the apple and fold into the mixture.

Spoon into silicone muffin cups and bake at 300 to 325° F for 25-30 minutes.

TIP:

This muffin batter can also be baked in a round silicone baking pan. Just leave out the chopped apples and spread natreen cherries or mandarin oranges on top. Bake as before.

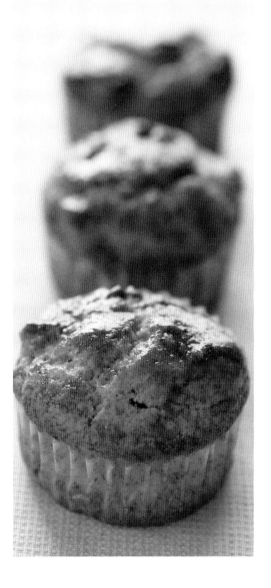

STABILIZATION AND TEST PHASE

Coconut Macaroons

Nutritional values

Approx. total
1922 kcal
(8074 kJ)
3.39 oz F
1.38 oz C
7.90 oz P

Ingredients:

2 oz	Protein powder 85 % vanilla or chocolate
2 oz	Whey protein 90 % vanilla or chocolate
1 tbsp	Cocoa powder
1	Egg
2	Egg whites
1 Cup	Water
2 oz	Almond flour
3 oz	Grated coconut
1 lb	Low fat Quark
3 oz	Sour cream 10 %
1 vial	Rum aroma or 1 tbsp rum
1 oz	Protein powder 85 % vanilla or coconut
	Ground vanilla

Preparation:

Blend the protein powder, whey protein, cocoa and water with hand mixer. Then add the egg, egg whites, 6 oz of the quark and the almond flour.

Next, spread the pastry dough (1 inch thick) in a rectangular silicone baking pan or on a baking tray lined with waxed paper. Place on the middle shelf of the oven and bake at 300 to 325 ° F for 15-20 minutes.

In the meantime, mix the rest of the quark, sour cream, grated coconut, rum or rum aroma, vanilla protein powder and ground vanilla and stir well.

After the macaroon base has cooled (do not worry about any air bubbles, as they will disappear) spread on the cream topping to about an inch thick and refrigerate for at least one hour.

TIP:

The pastry for the base can also be made just from protein powder and chocolate whey protein, 1 cup water, 4 oz quark and 3 egg whites. (With this method, air bubbles are very likely to appear. Once the base cools, however, they will disappear).

STABILIZATION AND TEST PHASE

Low Carb Poppy Seed Quark Pie

Ingredients:

3	Eggs
2 level tsp	Baking powder
1 level tsp	Guar meal
2 oz	Unflavored or vanilla protein powder
1 lb	Low fat Quark
7 oz	Ground poppy seeds
	Xylitol or Sukrin as desired

Nutritional values

Approx. total
1833 kcal
(7447 kJ)
3.74 oz F
1.55 oz C
6.38 oz P

Preparation:

Beat the eggs with a hand mixer until foamy and add the quark.

In a separate bowl, mix the protein powder with the baking powder and guar meal. Stir in the protein powder and xylitol or Sukrin to the egg/quark mixture to make a smooth batter. Lastly, add the ground poppy seeds.

Bake at 300 to 325 ° F for about 30 minutes. If the cake begins to brown too quickly, cover with waxed paper. Once baked, it is best to leave it for a few hours to allow the poppy seed flavor to develop.

Low Carb Quark Muffins

Ingredients:

6	Eggs
1 lb	Low fat Quark
1 lb	Ricotta
	Lemon aroma (health food shop)
	Liquid stevia or sucralose as desired
1 tbsp	Locust bean gum
2 tbsp	Rapeseed oil

Nutritional values

Approx. total
1930 kcal
(8093 kJ)
4.44 oz F
0.92 oz C
6.07 oz P

Preparation:

Mix ingredients in an electric food processor until you have a smooth batter. Spoon into silicone muffin cups and bake in a pre-heated fan oven at 300º F (middle shelf) for about 30 minutes. Open the oven and allow to cool.

STABILIZATION AND TEST PHASE

Low Carb Chocolate Cream Cake

Ingredients:

Batter:

5 oz	Chocolate flavored whey protein
4 tsp	Baking powder
2-1/2 oz	Cocoa powder
1 Cup	Water
4	Eggs

Cream:

1lb	Low fat Quark
2-1/2 oz	Vanilla flavored whey protein
2 tbsp	Locust bean gum
	Xylitol or Sukrin as desired

Nutritional values

Approx. total
1827 kcal
(7662 kJ)
1.52 oz F
1.87 oz C
10.86 oz P

Preparation:

Beat the ingredients for the batter with a hand mixer until smooth.

Spread evenly over a baking tray lined with waxed paper. Bake in a fan oven at 300 ° F for about 10 minutes and set aside to cool. Now cut in half.

Next mix the ingredients for the cream. Spread the cream on one half of the cake for the bottom layer and spread the remainder on the second half and place on top.

Low Carb Chocolate Cake

Ingredients:

2	Eggs
1 heaped tbsp	Gluten
2 oz	Protein powder
2 oz	Soy flour
3 tbsp	Cocoa powder
2 oz	Rapeseed oil
2 tsp	Baking powder
2/3 Cup	Milk
	Xylitol or Sukrin as desired

Nutritional values

Approx. total
1250 kcal
(5001 kJ)
3.03 oz F
0.88 oz C
3.56 oz P

Preparation:

In a bowl, beat together all the ingredients. Note: the batter will be very stiff.

Grease a mini 4 inch bundt pan or use a silicone baking pan and "flour" with cocoa powder. Spoon in the batter and bake in a fan oven at 300 to 325° F for about 30 minutes.

These amounts are for a 4 inch mini bundt pan. For larger cakes, simply adjust the amounts accordingly. Baking time will also be longer (test with a skewer). If you like, you can sift more cocoa powder over the cake.

STABILIZATION AND TEST PHASE

Ricotta Peanut Muffins

Nutritional values

Approx. total
2169 kcal
(9085 kJ)
5.36 oz F
1.83 oz C
5.22 oz P

Ingredients for 12 muffins:

9 oz	Ricotta
5 oz	Buttermilk
2	Eggs
4 oz	Peanut flour
3 oz	Protein powder
3 tblsp	Rapeseed oil
1 heaped tsp	Baking powder
1 large	Apple
	Peanuts, whole

Preparation:

Beat the ricotta, buttermilk and eggs until foamy. Then add the peanut flour, protein powder, rapeseed oil and baking powder.

Chop the apple and stir into the batter. Spoon into silicone muffin cups and garnish with the peanuts.

Bake the muffins in a fan oven at 300 to 325º F for about 30 minutes.

SWEET TREATS

Low Carb Chia Jam

Nutritional values

Approx. total
105 kcal
(438 kJ)
0.18 oz F
0.35 oz C
0.18 oz P

Ingredients:

3 tbsp	Chia seeds
9 oz	Rhubarb or another fruit
	Stevia or xylitol or Sukrin, as desired
	Cinnamon
	Water

Preparation:

Peel and cut the rhubarb into small pieces.

Simmer in a little water with cinnamon and a little stevia, xylitol or Sukrin until the rhubarb falls apart. Purée the fruit and add more of the natural sweeteners or cinnamon, if needed.

Lastly, add the chia seeds and spoon the jam into sterile jars. The chia seeds will act as pectin and make the jam set.

STABILIZATION AND TEST PHASE

Low Carb Coconut Pancakes

Nutritional values

Approx. total
528 kcal
(2491 kJ)
1.66 oz F
0.32 oz C
1.27 oz P

Ingredients:

2 tbsp	Low fat Quark
2	Eggs
1 tsp	Baking powder
3 tbsp	Grated coconut
1 tbsp	Protein powder
	Stevia or xylitol
2-3 tbsp	Coconut milk

Preparation:

Mix all the ingredients until smooth. Brush a non-stick pan with some oil and cook the pancakes.

Serve with fresh berries or other fruit or with quark with fruit.

Low Carb Mousse au Chocolat

Nutritional values

Approx. total
568 kcal
(2377 kJ)
1.38 oz F
1.09 oz C
0.88 oz P

Ingredients:

2 oz	Dark chocolate (80-99 %)
1/2 tsp	Instant coffee powder
3	Egg whites
2 oz	Low fat Quark
	Xylitol or Sukrin

Preparation:

Break the chocolate into pieces and melt in the microwave or a bain marie. Next, stir in the instant coffee.

Beat the egg whites with a pinch of salt until stiff. Stir the quark into the melted chocolate until smooth. Sweeten with xylitol or Sukrin to taste.

Carefully fold in the egg whites.

Spoon into two dessert dishes, cover and refrigerate for 2 hours.

STABILIZATION AND TEST PHASE

Low Carb Pancakes

Ingredients:

Version 1:

2-3	Eggs
1-2 tsp	Locust bean gum
2 tbsp	Xylitol or Sukrin
1 pinch	Baking powder
	Ground vanilla

Nutritional values

Approx. total
370 kcal
(1550 kJ)
0.88 oz F
0.88 oz C
0.70 oz P

Version 2:

1 tbsp	Butter, melted in microwave
1 tbsp	Vanilla flavored protein powder
3 tbsp	Water
1	Egg
	Xylitol or Sukrin

Nutritional values

Approx. total
392 kcal
(1641 kJ)
1.13 oz F
0.42 oz C
0.70 oz P

Version 3:

6-1/2 tbsp	Cream
1 cup	Water
3	Eggs
	Xylitol or Sukrin, as desired
5 tbsp	Almond flour
2 1/2 tsp	Locust bean gum

Nutritional values

Approx. total
968 kcal
(4059 kJ)
3.07 oz F
0.60 oz C
1.31 oz P

Preparation:

For all versions, beat the ingredients together with an electric hand mixer, making sure the batter does not become lumpy.

Fry in a little butter until golden brown.

STABILIZATION AND TEST PHASE

Protein Nut Bar

Ingredients:

4 tsp	Protein powder, e.g. chocolate
4 tsp	Unsweetened peanut butter
2 tsp	Cocoa powder
2/3 cup	Linseed flour
1/4 cup	Water

Nutritional values

Approx. total
580 kcal
(2427 kJ)
1.16 oz F
0.32 oz C
2.19 oz P

Preparation:

Beat all the ingredients together until smooth. Shape into bars and wrap in plastic. Refrigerate until firm.

Vanilla Pancakes

Ingredients:

3	Egg whites
4 tbsp	Vanilla protein powder
3 tbsp	Psyllium husks
4 tbsp	Water

Nutritional values

Approx. total
245 kcal
(1024 kJ)
0.04 oz F
0.14 oz C
1.45 oz P

Preparation:

Beat all the ingredients together with an electric hand mixer and set aside for 5 minutes. Spoon the batter into the molds of a pancake maker.

Avocado Parmesan Butter

Ingredients:

9 oz	Softened salted butter
1	Very ripe avocado
3.5 oz	Grated Parmesan
	Salt, pepper, rosemary

Nutritional values

Approx. total
2680 kcal
(11219 kJ)
9.98 oz F
0.18 oz C
1.34 oz P

Preparation:

Mash the avocado with the butter and mix in some grated Parmesan cheese. Season with salt, pepper and rosemary to taste. Enjoy!

Chinese Cabbage/Bok Choi au gratin

Ingredients:

2 lbs	Chinese Cabbage/Bok Choi
4-1/2 oz	Gorgonzola
2-1/2 oz	Whipping cream
1/2 cup	Whole milk
	Butter for the casserole dish

Nutritional values

Approx. total
959 kcal
(4001 kJ)
2.79 oz F
0.67 oz C
1.34 oz P

Preparation:

Pre-heat the oven to 350° F (fan 325° F). Remove outer leaves of the Chinese Cabbage/Bok Choi. Cut into dice, wash carefully and shake dry. Beat together the Gorgonzola, cream and the milk until creamy.

Lightly grease a casserole dish. Place the cabbage into the dish and cover evenly with the gorgonzola cream. Bake on the middle shelf for about 25 minutes. Salt and pepper to taste.

TIP:

Belgian endives or radicchio taste very good as well if baked in this way. For a more pungent dish, you can substitute the Gorgonzola with Roquefort.

Low Carb Mozzarella Pizza

Nutritional values
Approx. total
2665 kcal
(11158 kJ)
3.28 oz F
0.88 oz C
7.16 oz P

Ingredients:

1-1/4 lbs	Mozzarella
4 oz	Freshly grated Parmesan cheese
4 oz	Low fat cream cheese
2 oz	Whipping cream
3	Eggs
1 can	Chopped tomatoes
	Salt, pepper, pizza spices
1	Bell pepper
4-5	Mushrooms
2 oz	Smoked turkey breast

Preparation:

Brush a baking tray with oil. Spread a thick layer of finely sliced mozzarella, reserving any left over for the topping.

Whisk the cream cheese, eggs and Parmesan and pour over the mozzarella. Bake the pizza base in a fan oven at 350° F for about 30 minutes.

Remove from the oven and top with seasoned tomato pieces, bell pepper strips, mushrooms, diced turkey breast and any left-over mozzarella. Bake for about 10-15 minutes more until golden brown.

BREADS

Low Carb Chickpea Bread

Nutritional values
Approx. total
(without grain)
1840 kcal
(7707 kJ)
4.55 oz F
3.32 oz C
2.82 oz P

Ingredients:

1-3/4 cups	Chickpea flour
4 oz	Butter
5	Eggs
1 tsp	Salt
1-1/2 tbsp	Baking powder
	Linseeds, sunflower seeds, nuts
	(Variety and amount of your choice)

Preparation:

Separate the eggs and beat the whites until stiff. Beat the yolks, butter, chickpea flour, baking powder, salt and seeds/nuts until smooth. Fold in the egg whites.

Pour the mixture into a silicone baking pan and bake at 300 to 325° F for about 45 minutes.

Sweet Coconut Bread

Ingredients (for 12 slices)

3-1/2 oz	Coconut flour
6	Eggs
4 oz	Soft butter
1 tsp	Baking powder
2 tsp	Xylitol or Sukrin
1/2 tsp	Salt

Preparation:

Cream the butter, eggs, xylitol or Sukrin.

Add the remaining ingredients little by little until you have a smooth dough.

Place in a silicone baking pan and bake in a fan oven at 300 to 325° F for 40 to 45 minutes.

Nutritional values

Approx. total
1754 kcal
(7349 kJ)
5.11 oz F
2.12 oz C
2.19 oz P

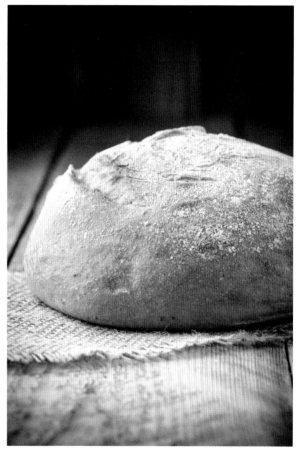

Low Carb Berry Pie

Nutritional values
Approx. total
2961 kcal
(12405 kJ)
7.37 oz F
5.08 oz C
4.20 oz P

Ingredients:

For the Pastry:

5	Eggs
4-1/2 oz	Xylitol or Sukrin
1 cup	Whole milk
2 bars (6 oz)	Dark chocolate, minimum 80 %
4 oz	Coconut flour
1/2 tbsp	Baking powder

For the Filling:

7 oz	Low fat quark
1 cup	Whipping cream
6 tbsp	Xylitol or Sukrin
10-1/2 oz	Berries

Preparation:

Grease a round 7" baking pan. Pre-heat the oven to 325° F (fan).

Beat the eggs and xylitol or Sukrin for at least 8 minutes. Next, melt the chocolate slowly in the microwave. Pour the milk into the egg mixture. Next mix the coconut flour with the baking powder. Now incorporate the melted chocolate into the egg mixture and stir well. Sift the coconut flour and fold in carefully.

Pour into the baking pan and bake for about 50 minutes. Check with a skewer to see if done.

Slice the cake through the middle to form two layers and set aside to cool.

Whip the cream with the xylitol or Sukrin until stiff and fold in the quark.

Spread the filling on to the bottom layer of cake and cover with berries. Spread another thin layer of filling on top of the berries and cover with the top layer of cake. If desired, spread more of the cream filling on the top and decorate with all kinds of berries.

Low Carb Cheese Cake

Ingredients:

Base:

2 cups	Almond flour
4-1/2 oz	Butter
1	Egg
3 oz	Xylitol or Sukrin

Filling:

2 lbs	Greek yoghurt
6	Eggs
	Xylitol or Sukrin, optional
	Cinnamon, lemon, rum or almond essence, as desired

Nutritional values

Approx. total
4166 kcal
(17447 kJ)
13.51 oz F
1.87 oz C
4.90 oz P

Preparation:

Knead all the ingredients together for the base and press into a spring form pan. (It will not be possible to roll out as there is no gluten).

Mix the Greek yoghurt with the eggs, xylitol or Sukrin and add the flavoring of your choice, if desired.

Spread the yoghurt filling evenly over the base.

Bake in a fan oven for 1 – 1-1/2 hours at 300 to 325° F until golden brown.

TEST PHASE

Low Carb Raspberry Roll

Nutritional values
Approx. total
1107 kcal
(4638 kJ)
3.49 oz F
0.70 oz C
1.34 oz P

Ingredients:

For the Sponge:

3	Eggs
1	Egg yolk
5 tbsp	Xylitol or Sukrin
1-1/2 tbsp	Coconut flour
1 tbsp	Grated coconut
1 tsp	Baking powder

Filling:

1 cup	Whipping cream
3 tbsp	Xylitol or Sukrin
2 oz	Raspberries, puréed

Preparation:

Pre-heat a fan oven to 300° F. Line a baking tray with waxed paper.

Mix the eggs with xylitol or Sukrin and beat until foamy (about 8 minutes). Mix the coconut flour with the grated coconut and the baking powder and add to the egg mixture, stirring well to incorporate. Pour the batter on to the baking tray and bake for about 12 minutes.

Next you will need two tea towels – one wet and one dry. With the dry towel on the table, turn the sponge cake out, paper side up. Now place the wet towel on top of the waxed paper. This will help to loosen the sponge more easily. As soon as the waxed paper has been completely removed, using the towel, roll up the sponge and set aside to cool.

In the meantime, puree the raspberries and sweeten to taste.

Beat the whipping cream with the xylitol or Sukrin until stiff, fold in the raspberries.

Unroll the sponge and cover with a layer of the filling. Roll up again carefully.

Low Carb Raspberry Cake

Nutritional values

Approx. total
2639 kcal
(11062 kJ)
7.05 oz F
2.19 oz C
5.29 oz P

Ingredients:

For the base:

3 oz	Butter
4	Eggs
1-1/2 cups	Ground almonds
1/2 cup	Whipping cream or milk
1 vial	Vanilla butter essence
	Xylitol or Sukrin, optional
3/4 tbsp	Baking powder

Cream for the topping

9 oz	Raspberries (fresh or frozen)
1 sachet	Cake glaze
	Xylitol or Sukrin as desired
6 sheets	Gelatin
1 lb	Low fat quark
1 tbsp	Lemon juice
1 cup	Cream (or low fat quark in addition to the 1 lb)

Preparation:

Separate the eggs and beat the whites until stiff. Beat together the butter, ground almonds, egg yolks, vanilla butter essence, baking powder, xylitol or Sukrin and cream. Lastly, carefully fold in the egg whites.

Spoon the batter into a round baking pan lined with waxed paper and bake at 350° F for about 30 minutes

Defrost and purée the berries. Mix the cake glaze with xylitol or Sukrin. Then add the puréed berries. Bring to a boil in a saucepan, stirring continuously. Set aside to cool.

In the meantime, follow the directions for soaking the gelatin in water and squeeze out slightly. In a saucepan, taking care not to let it boil, warm the gelatin mixture until it is completely dissolved. Add a little water, if needed.

Next mix the quark with the xylitol or Sukrin and lemon juice. Stir about 4 tbsp of the quark mixture into the gelatin and then incorporate the remainder. As soon as it begins to set, whip the cream into stiff peaks and fold into the quark filling.

Now alternately layer the quark filling and then the berry purée on to the base finishing with a layer of the quark. Marble slightly with the back of a spoon. Then refrigerate for 2 hours. Remove the cake carefully from the form.

TEST PHASE

Low Carb Orange Cake

Ingredients:

9	Eggs
9 tbsp	Xylitol or Sukrin
6 oz	Coconut flour
5-1/4 oz	Butter, melted
3 cups	Freshly squeezed orange juice
1-1/2 tbsp	Baking powder

Nutritional values

Approx. total
3032 kcal
(12697 kJ)
7.59 oz F
5.78 oz C
3.88 oz P

Preparation:

Pre-heat a fan oven to 300° F.

Beat the eggs with xylitol or Sukrin for at least 5 minutes until foamy. Next add 2 cups of orange juice and the melted butter. Mix the baking powder with the coconut flour and incorporate. Pour the batter into a round silicone baking pan or into a greased baking pan.

Bake the cake for about 30 minutes. Set aside to cool. Prick the cake with a fork and drizzle with the remaining orange juice.

Low Carb Russian Chocolate Cheesecake

Ingredients:

For the base:

5-1/4 oz	Butter, melted
14 oz	Ground almonds
1-1/2 oz	Oat bran
5 oz	Vanilla or unflavored protein powder
5 tbsp	Xylitol or Sukrin
7 tbsp	Unsweetened cocoa powder
4	Eggs
4 tsp	Baking powder

Nutritional values

Approx. total
5415 kcal
(22712 kJ)
15.10 oz F
2.36 oz C
11.85 oz P

Filling:

9 oz	Low fat quark
2	Eggs
3 tbsp	Vanilla protein powder
1 tbsp	Locust bean gum

Preparation:

Beat the melted butter with the eggs until foamy. Incorporate the dry ingredients a little at a time until a dough is formed. Gently press a little more than half of the dough into a round 10" silicone baking pan. Next, mix together the ingredients for the filling and spread on to the base. Lastly, crumble over the remaining dough to make a topping.

Bake in a fan oven at 300 to 325° F for 60 – 65 minutes.

Low Carb Chocolate Cake

Ingredients:

9	Eggs
3 oz	Coconut flour
5-1/4 oz	Butter, melted
5-1/4 oz	Xylitol or Sukrin
1-1/2 tbsp	Baking powder
3 oz	Unsweetened cocoa powder

Nutritional values

Approx. total
2263 kcal
(11025 kJ)
7.58 oz F
2.36 oz C
3.63 oz P

Preparation:

Pre-heat a fan oven to 300° F. Grease a 5" spring form pan with butter or use a silicone baking pan.

Beat the eggs and xylitol or Sukrin until foamy (about 5 minutes). Next, melt the butter and beat into the eggs. Mix together the coconut flour, cocoa and baking powder and incorporate quickly into the other ingredients. Spoon the thick batter into the spring form pan and bake for about 25 minutes. When checking to see if the cake is done, it is fine if the toothpick does not come out completely clean.

Low Carb Chocolate Muffins

Ingredients:

4	Eggs
8 tbsp	Flax seeds, ground
4 tbsp	Cottage cheese
1 cup	Whipping Cream
8 tbsp	Melted butter
12 tbsp	Cocoa powder
4 tbsp	Sukrin or xylitol

Nutritional values

Approx. total
3047 kcal
(12764 kJ)
9.38 oz F
1.31 oz C
4.80 oz P

Preparation:

Pre-heat a fan oven to 300 – 325° F. Mix together all the ingredients and spoon into silicone muffin cups. Bake for 20-30 minutes. Set aside to cool before removing from the muffin cups.

TEST PHASE

Low Carb Chocolate Roll

Nutritional values

Approx. total	1100 kcal
	(4611 kJ)
3.28 oz	F
0.67 oz	C
1.45 oz	P

Ingredients:

For the sponge:

3	Eggs
1	Egg yolk
5 tbsp	Xylitol or Sukrin
1-1/2 tbsp	Coconut flour
1-1/2 tbsp	Unsweetened cocoa powder/Baking chocolate powder
1/2 tbsp	Baking powder

Cream:

1 cup	Whipping cream
3 tbsp	Xylitol or Sukrin
1/2 tbsp	Unsweetened cocoa powder/baking chocolate powder

Preparation:

Pre-heat a fan oven to 300 – 325° F. Line a baking tray with waxed paper.

Mix the eggs with the xylitol or Sukrin and beat until foamy (about 8 minutes). Mix the coconut flour with the cocoa and baking powder and add to the batter. Stir again well. Bake for about 12 minutes.

Now you will need two tea towels, one of them wet. Spread the dry one on the table and place the sponge cake on the towel with the waxed paper facing up. Now place the wet towel on top of the waxed paper. This way, the sponge will loosen easily from the paper. Then, with the help of the dry towel, roll up the sponge cake and set aside to cool.

Whip the cocoa powder and cream with the xylitol or Sukrin until stiff.

Unroll the cooled sponge, spread the whipped cream over it and then carefully roll back up.

Low Carb Swedish Almond Cake

Nutritional values

Approx. total
3009 kcal
(12607 kJ)
10.30 oz F
0.60 oz C
3.25 oz P

Ingredients:

For the cake:

6	Egg whites
7 oz	Ground almonds
3 – 4 oz	Xylitol or Sukrin

Cream:

3 – 4 oz	Xylitol or Sukrin
1 cup	Whipping cream
4 oz	Butter, softened
6	Egg yolks

Preparation:

Pre-heat a fan oven to 300 – 325º F. Grease either a spring form pan with butter or use a silicone baking pan. Separate the eggs. Beat the egg whites with the xylitol or Sukrin (sweeten to taste) until stiff. Carefully fold in the ground almonds.

Spoon the batter into the pan and bake for about 30 min. Set aside to cool completely.

In the meantime, bring the whipping cream to a boil with the xylitol or Sukrin. Remove the saucepan from the heat and, using an electric hand mixer, beat in the egg yolks. Re-heat the cream, stirring continuously. Set aside to cool. Add the softened butter to the cream and beat again until creamy.

Ice the cake with the cream. If desired, toast a handful of almonds in a pan and sprinkle over the cake for decoration.

SWEET TREATS

Low Carb Chocolate Cream

Nutritional values

Approx. total
1210 kcal
(5065 kJ)
4.30 oz F
0.63 oz C
0.53 oz P

Ingredients:

4 oz	Whipping cream
2 tbsp	Unsweetened cocoa powder/baking chocolate powder
2-1/2 oz	Freshly ground hazelnuts
2-1/2 oz	Melted butter
1-2 tsp	Ground Cinnamon
1 tsp	Ground vanilla
1-2 tsp	Xylitol or Sukrin

Preparation:

Melt the butter in the microwave for about 1 minute at 800 watts. Next incorporate the remaining ingredients stirring vigorously with a fork. Pour the chocolate cream into a jar and refrigerate. (Its shelf life is about 3-4 days). This tastes very good on LOGI Bread or LOGI Rolls (LOGI= Low Glycemic Index).

Delicious Low Carb Nut Candy

	Nutritional values
	Approx. total
	1829 kcal
	(7661 kJ)
	6.74 oz F
	0.42 oz C
	0.81 oz P

Ingredients:

1	Egg
1/4 cup	Whipping cream
3 tsp	Hazelnut flour
4 tsp	Unsweetened cocoa powder, baking chocolate powder
1/2 tsp	Vanilla, ground
	Xylitol or Sukrin
5 oz	Coconut oil
	Chopped walnuts

Preparation:

Beat the first 6 ingredients with an electric hand mixer until smooth. The cocoa powder should no longer be lumpy.

Warm up the coconut oil (not too hot) and, on a low speed, beat into the batter.

Next spoon the batter into a silicone ice tray, decorate with the chopped walnuts and freeze for about 30 minutes.

Fluffy Low Carb Pancakes

	Nutritional values
	Approx. total
	1231 kcal
	(5154 kJ)
	3.95 oz F
	0.21 oz C
	1.87 oz P

Ingredients:

4 oz	Butter
	Xylitol or Sukrin
2	Eggs
1 pinch	Salt
3 tbsp	Vanilla protein powder
1-2 drops	Lemon juice
2 oz	Full fat sour cream or Quark

Preparation:

Cream the butter. Add the remaining ingredients and mix well. Bake in a pan on a low heat. Add more xylitol or Sukrin powder if desired.

To save calories, use less butter and Quark instead of full fat sour cream.

The batter can also be used for making waffles (1 heaped spoonful for a waffle).

Low Carb Waffles

Ingredients (makes about 10 square waffles)

8	Eggs
4-1/2 oz	Butter, melted
7 oz	Low fat Quark
4 tsp	Rapeseed oil
2 tsp	Baking powder
4-1/2 oz	Vanilla or coconut protein powder
	Cinnamon, ground vanilla, as desired

Nutritional values

Approx. total
2397 kcal
(10045 kJ)
6.17 oz F
0.92 oz C
6.49 oz P

Preparation:

Cream the eggs and the melted butter with an electric hand mixer. Add the remaining ingredients little by little and set aside for 5 minutes to rise.

Cook in a non-stick waffle pan.

TIP:

This same batter can also be made with grated cheese and diced ham. Use unflavored protein powder and, instead of cinnamon and vanilla, season with pepper.

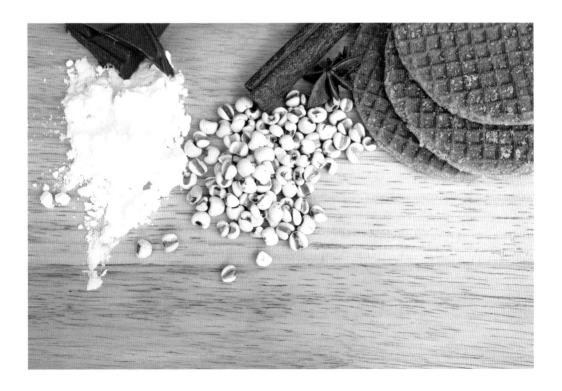

FAQs – Questions and Answers

With every new situation, there is always an element of insecurity. The 21 Day Metabolic Diet is just such a new situation because you will notice many changes in yourself. Naturally this will raise questions. We have compiled the most frequently asked questions for you but, of course, there are many more.

Because it is important to us that you feel comfortable, if you are not sure about something, please do not hesitate to ask your health consultant or sponsor. They will be able to answer any specific questions or needs you might have.

Headaches during the metabolic diet

Question: What can I do if I suffer from headaches at the beginning or during the diet?

Answer: Especially at the beginning of the Metabolic Diet, you may experience headaches because the body has to adapt to something completely new. It may be the case, depending on the initial circumstances that a large amount of toxins are released into the body and these now need to be flushed out. To remedy this, drink lots of still water and take organic sulfur. You may also wish to add chlorella or some goat's whey into your lunch. If necessary, a gentle headache remedy can also bring fast relief.

Something is taking place in your body, so do not resort too quickly to painkillers. It is better to flush out the toxins.

Dieting without losing weight?

Question: Does it make sense to do this diet if I only want to do something good for my body without losing weight?

Answer: In short, yes, however in a modified way. The caloric intake must be balanced. This means a low carb diet should be maintained while the protein intake should not exceed a healthy amount (a rule of thumb is 1-1/4 oz pure protein per meal, depending on age, gender and muscle mass) and the remaining calories should come from high-quality fats. In this case, the energetic activator will not be necessary. The Metabolic Diet can also help you to improve the actual composition of your body and thus your wellbeing without weight loss.

Lactose intolerance

Question: I suffer from lactose intolerance. Are there any alternatives to the shake in the morning?

Answer: In this case, you should choose a protein isolate. Since it provides an unprecedented blend of superior sources of protein in isolate form, it is also suitable for those who are lactose intolerant.

Prescription Medication

Question: I would like to do the Metabolic Diet, however, at the moment I am taking prescription medication. Can I still do it?

Answer: Basically, taking prescription medication will not prevent you from being successful with the diet. The body metabolizes each medicine in a different way. Every change also leads to a variation in the metabolism. This is something you and your prescribing doctor need to be prepared for. This also means you should make more frequent check-ups to ensure you can respond appropriately to any changes in the body. What is more, you should be able to reduce the strength of your prescription medication or even stop it altogether! So, it is better to be upfront with your doctor. For best results, my advice is to have a clear channel of communication with your doctor, regular check-ups and make appropriate adjustments, as and when needed.

Eggs and dairy products during the diet phase

Question: Why should I not eat eggs or dairy products during the diet phase if I am not a vegetarian?

Answer: The concept of the diet has been developed to ensure maximum success. Any deviation from the instructions may mean poorer results.

After you have finished the diet phase, eggs and dairy products can be included again in your daily menu.

Choice of vegetables / salads during the diet phase

Question: Can I eat other vegetables and types of salad during the diet phase?

Answer: The list of approved foods has been tried and tested a million times by those who have done the diet successfully. Those who deviate from this list are entering uncharted waters. However, everyone has to decide for themselves if they prefer to stick to the tried and tested way or instead deviate from it by expanding their choice of vegetables / salads with other varieties with a low glycemic index.

Vegetarians, vegans

Question: What alternatives do I have with regard to sources of protein if I am a vegetarian or vegan?

Answer: Abstaining from meat hardly has any impact on the outcome of the diet. If you are vegetarian, eggs, low fat cheese (such as Harzer cheese) and tofu are recommended as they contain lots of high-quality protein. Tofu provides the best source of protein for vegans and can be eaten in any form. In the recipe part of the book you will find ideas for delicious vegan meals.

Plateaux and extension of the low calorie phase of the diet

Question: What can I do if I do not lose weight during longer periods?

Answer: Your body is not a machine. Metabolic processes do not run regularly like trains but rather in alternating periods of activity and rest. This does not mean, however, that nothing is happening to your body when you do not lose weight for a couple of days. Your body composition is still changing. It just may not be visible at that moment. If you are very impatient, then include an apple day in your diet. For one day eat only six tart apples in addition to your supplements. However, it would be better if you simply remained patient and kept to the diet plan.

Question: Can I extend the low calorie phase beyond 42 days?

Answer: Basically, yes. As we see it and from our experience, there is no reason why not, but you should still consult your doctor for the green light. Should he advise you to take a break, then start with the stabilization phase. After the stabilization phase and a break of at least 6-8 weeks, you can begin another low calorie diet phase.

Oral Contraception and the Metabolic Diet

Question: I am taking birth control. Is there anything I have to consider during the diet?

Answer: From the medical point of view, the "pill" as it is often referred to, comprises primarily two completely different medications: there is either the combined pill consisting of a combination of estrogen and progesterone or a progesterone-only "minipill". Both contraceptive pills have differing effects and reliability (expressed as the Pearl-Index i.e. the number of unwanted pregnancies in 100 women per year who use this form of contraception).

Basically, a subtle acting agent (energetically activated, homeopathic, radionic) will not neutralize a chemical reaction in the body. Neither does the activator with subtle effect during the 21 day metabolic diet. Therefore, the birth control pill is considered to be safe.

However (in terms of everyday life) we cannot exclude, let alone measure, the physiological sensitivity to certain hormonal changes while taking such gentle preparations. We also see the positive effects such as not feeling hungry, the change in the set-point, and so forth.

Before you start the metabolic diet, you should inform your gynecologist and ask for their advice as far as other contraceptive methods are concerned during the diet.

Atopic Dermatitis

Question: I am suffering from atopic dermatitis. What could happen to my skin during the diet?

Answer: During the diet, the body releases an increased amount of toxins. Together with the kidneys, intestines and lungs, the skin is also an organ that eliminates toxins from the body. In some cases, it is possible that, at the beginning of the diet, any skin condition could worsen. After a few days, however, we mostly see that the body adjusts and the skin improves. If you are not sure about this, then do not hesitate to ask your doctor. An experienced practitioner can explain any underlying issues and offer you help during the initial phase.

Stubborn cellulitis that never goes away or only goes away very slowly?

Question: I had a fantastic result with the diet in reference to weight loss. However, I would like to do more for my cellulitis. What can I do?

Answer: The improvement of the connective tissue simply takes longer than the weight reduction. First of all, you need to be patient. You must continuously provide your body with micronutrients (antioxidants) and organic sulfur. Furthermore, it is important to maintain your acid-alkaline (pH) balance (e.g. with alkaline baths, alkaline teas or tablets). Do sports, e.g. fitness training, Nordic walking or swimming. Regular brush massages in the evenings are recommended for stimulating the blood supply to the connective tissue.

Diabetes and the 21 Day Metabolic Diet

Question: I am a diabetic. What specific issues do I need to consider?

Answer: Basically, diabetes should not pose a problem to having good results with the metabolic diet. However, depending on your individual type of treatment, it may be necessary to work closely with your physician. If you are able to manage your blood sugar levels through your diet, there will be no need for further action. However should you be on medication, then a new, personalized treatment should be established together with your doctor or diabetes specialist. At first, this may entail a little more effort and control, but afterwards your metabolic condition will have significantly improved. And that is what counts. So, in any event, if you are diabetic, consult your physician before you start the metabolic diet.

Blood Thinners and the 21 Day Metabolic Diet

Question: I would like to do the metabolic diet but I am on blood thinners (e.g. Warfarin/Coumadin). What special issues do I need to consider?

Answer: As a rule, you should consult your physician before you begin the metabolic diet. There are some blood thinners that do not require any further action, however there are others that need to be carefully adjusted and monitored. Since every

change in your body influences your metabolism, the dose has to be strictly monitored and adjusted if necessary. So, do not hesitate to discuss this with your physician and get checked frequently for any adjustments to your medication. It´s worth it!

Young People and the 21 Day Metabolic Diet

Question: My son/daughter would like to do the diet. From what age can this diet be recommended?

Answer: As a rule, young people from the age of 16 can go on the diet. For anyone younger, it should be decided whether it is appropriate on an individual basis. In these circumstances, their GP should be consulted before getting started. The goal may be to eat healthily, provide their bodies with sufficient micronutrients and organic sulfur to flush out toxins, and to monitor their pH balance. The use of an energetic activator is only recommended for adults. In principle, it is important that this is something they want to do for themselves and not considered a punishment from their parents.

Sports and the 21 Day Metabolic Diet

Question: I want to do sports or keep my sports activities up during the diet. Is there anything special I have to consider?

Answer: During the low calorie phase your body is supplied with sufficient energy from its own body fat. From our experience, there is no loss of physical performance during the diet phase. Monitor your body carefully and give yourself some time as it has to adjust to a completely new situation. Depending on the initial circumstances, a large amount of toxins may have to be eliminated and this change will mean an additional strain on the body. Many participants report that, after this initial phase their physical condition improved and that they feel "fitter" when doing sports.

Counteracting a lack of energy during peak exertion

Question: I am doing a lot of sport. Since I have started the diet I feel a little tired.

Answer: When doing a lot of sport you might feel a loss of energy during physical exertion or maximum cognitive performance. In this case there is nothing wrong with having an aspartame free protein shake in between meals.

Our clients love a drink with Arginin from Lifeplus. It tastes delicious, provides energy, promotes the building of muscles and increases circulation.

Tip: Mix the shake in the morning with a sugar-free vitamin drink or (as a concession) with some freshly squeezed orange juice.

Thyroid and the 21 Day Metabolic Diet

Question: What special issues need to be considered when someone has thyroid problems or has had their thyroid removed?

Answer: If you have an underlying case of hyperthyroidism, do not add iodine to your diet. So, check your supplements for iodine. You may want to show them to your physician. (The drink that contains minerals, vitamins and fiber without iodine). Should you take medication for your thyroid, you will want to make a note of any changes. Get regular checks-ups and adjust the dose of your medication as necessary. However, this should not pose a problem.

Sweeteners

Question: Are there alternatives for common sugar?

Answer: Stevia (also called candy leaf or sweet honey leaf) is a sweet-tasting plant native to South America which is processed into a healthy sweetener in many countries. Stevia does not contain any calories or sugar.

The concentrated sweetness extracted from stevia is called stevioside and is 300 times sweeter than common sugar. Stevia can even be used during the low calorie phase of the diet.

If you like to bake with stevia you may want to consider recipes that have been especially elaborated for its use.

The xylitol (birch sugar) mentioned in the recipes is an alternative for stevia. Sukrin, a premium brand for the sugar alcohol Erythritol can also be used as a substitute.

Sukrin is 100 % natural. Amongst other things, it can be found in ripe fruits such as melons, pears and grapes. It has been consumed from time immemorial in small quantities. Fermented foods like cheese, wine and soy sauce also contain Sukrin. Furthermore, Sukrin is present in the human body and is very well tolerated.

Sukrin is made from glucose which is natural. The structure of the sugar changes by means of a process of fermentation, similar to that of ripening fruits or cheese. For this procedure they use containers such as those in breweries. The result is a completely natural product: the sugar alcohol Erythritol, produced from common sugar or glucose. After putting it through an elaborate crystallization process and a special quality control, Sukrin is produced.

After thorough examination, Sukrin was approved by the European Union in 2006. In Japan it received approval as early as 1990 and in the USA it has been on the market since 1997. When compared to other sugar alcohols, Sukrin is noticeably smaller. The other sugar alcohols such as xylitol, due to their size, are not absorbed in the small intestine. They travel further on to the colon where they are broken down into small fatty molecules and stored by the body as energy (calories). They also cause a higher osmotic pressure in the colon: that is the difference in concentration between the colon and its surroundings. The body tries to offset this difference in concentration by releasing water into the bowel. This leads to an expansion of the walls of the colon which can have a laxative effect.

Sukrin, however, is absorbed in the small intestine and thus does not cause any significant digestive issues. The body does not turn Sukrin into energy. It is instead excreted into the urine and for this reason is the only calorie free sugar alcohol.

It does not have to be counted as bread units or carbohydrates and is therefore ideal for diabetics and anyone who wants to eat a low-calorie diet.

Bodycare products during the Metabolic Diet

Question: Do I have to stop using my usual body care products?

Answer: If you want to lose as much weight as possible, then you should not use products that contain oils or fats during the low calorie phase of the diet. During that period substitute your usual skin care with moisturizing products such as aloe vera gel.

Food intolerances

Question: What can I eat if I am fructose intolerant?

Answer: As a rule any food intolerances take priority. Leave out what you cannot tolerate. As far as fructose intolerance: for people with fructose intolerance the fructose content is not as important as the ratio of glucose to fructose.

As already mentioned on page 11, fruit should only be eaten if necessary but, if fructose intolerant, the following fruits may be eaten in small quantities:

Apricots, blackberries, grapefruit, raspberries, honeydew melon, lichees, tangerines, small yellow plums, nectarines.

Forgot to take the activator

Question: What do I have to do if I forgot to take the energetic activator?

Answer: Nothing – just continue with the program.

Minimum amount of liquids needed

Question: Why do I have to drink so much?

Answer: Our body is 60 % water. An adult loses about 2-1/2 quarts of water every day. As an average we absorb about 1 quart with our food and the rest by drinking. During the diet you need enough water to flush out the toxins e.g. through the urine. It is best to drink the liquids needed throughout the day. As a rule of thumb, you should drink 1 oz to 1-1/4 oz per 2 lbs body weight per day. Thus, a 175 lb person needs to consume between 2-1/2 to 3 quarts.

Quantity of protein

Question: Is the 21-Day Metabolic Diet a so-called "protein" diet?

Answer: During the 21-Day Metabolic Diet the daily intake of protein corresponds to 0.04 oz – 0.05 oz of protein per 2 lbs body weight, which is consumed as an average in Central Europe. This means 3 oz – 3-3/4 oz protein for a person weighing 165 lbs. The German Association for Nutrition (DGE) recommends a protein supply no higher than 0.07 oz per 2 lbs body weight.

Risks and side effects of energetic activators

Question: Is it safe to take energetic activators?

Answer: To date, there have been no drawbacks or side effects from taking the energetic activator reported by the over 500,000 people who have participated in the metabolic diet.

Alternative metabolic activators

Question: Are there any alternatives to energetic activators?

Answer: Yes, besides radionic globules, drops or salts, there are homeopathic products. The principle of transmission of information is similar in both cases. However, the method of transmission is significantly different and yet the success in both types of procedures is comparable.

Information for the attending physician

The Metabolic Diet supported by an energetic activator

The goal of the metabolic diet is for a lasting reduction in weight. It consists of 4 phases: 2 loading days, a minimum 21 day low calorie diet, a 21 day stabilization phase and a 6 month test phase.

For the 2 loading days please note the following:

➡ The participants intentionally stock up on carbohydrates

For this reason it is recommended that they eat food that is preferably high in fat and carbohydrates.

➡ After these 2 days, the actual diet phase begins.

For the 21 day diet phase, please note the following:

➡ The participants will follow a diet regime that involves a reduced caloric intake: three meals a day with low fat protein and plenty of vegetables and salad.

➡ The energetic activator is intended to target the stored body fat. Structural fat is not targeted, however dangerous visceral fat, in particular, will decrease.

➡ The body is provided with the energy it needs from the three meals and its own fat cells that are broken down.

At the same time your patients support their health with first class, absolutely natural nutritional supplements with no artificial additives.

Organic sulfur – for the detoxification of the body

➡ It increases the permeability of the cell membrane enabling the body to absorb more nutrients and to eliminate accumulated metabolic waste.

➡ It serves as a catalyst for vitamins and minerals

➡ It is an antioxidant. It deactivates toxins in the body and accelerates their elimination

➡ It relieves discomfort from allergies

➡ It increases the absorption of oxygen

➡ It increases absorption of cellular glucose in diabetics

➡ It relieves cramps and muscle pain

Antioxidant (OPCs) – cell protection and recovery of the skin

➡ OPCs (oligomeric proanthocyanidins) protect collagen and elastin and keep the skin elastic and smooth

➡ They activate and increase vitamin C tenfold and, by crossing the blood brain barrier, the brain cells are protected as well.

➡ Sagging skin becomes firm again

➡ Significantly improved and rejuvenated skin

➡ Internal and external cell protection

Please see: A. Simons and A. Rucker: "Living Longer in Good Health through OPCs"

Essential fatty acids

➡ Supply of the body with Omega-3 for a regulated ratio between Omega-3 and Omega-6 fatty acids

A nutritional drink that supplies the body with a comprehensive selection of vitamins, minerals, herbal extracts and fiber

➡ It also contains probiotics

For the stabilization phase please note the following:

➡ The caloric intake will now be increased to stabilize the weight

➡ The goal is to engage in a healthy life style on a long term basis

IN A NUTSHELL, the aim is for a healthy pH balance and a cleansed intestine. In addition, there is a clear focus on reducing the risk of cardio-vascular disease. Due to the positive effect of the diet on obesity, high blood pressure, increased lipid levels and diabetes mellitus type 2, this is entirely possible.

Where to buy

As mentioned in this book, my clients have had very positive experiences with the nutritional supplements from Lifeplus (www.lifeplus.com). You can also get the aspartame free protein shake for the Metabolic Diet from them. Should you use nutritional supplements from another company, please make sure you only buy high quality ones because the success of the diet depends on it (Please see page 14). Good quality has its price. You should thoroughly check to see if the nutritional supplements from the supermarket around the corner, offered for next to nothing, meet high quality standards. How many people would be happy to pay 5,000 euros or more if they knew that they would look better and feel healthier afterwards? If someone has recommended this book to you, then ask your sponsor for the appropriate products.

Activators for the Metabolic Diet can be bought over the internet. As mentioned before, there are a variety of activators. They can come in the form of globules, salts or drops. Actually, it makes no difference. All of them work and should be taken as an accompaniment to the Metabolic Diet. Here are a few providers of the activators:

➡ www.newvistashealthcare.com

➡ www.viteffect.de

➡ www.biovea.com